HEALING WITH CHINESE HERBS

夏瑴窯編著

中藥淺說

高山村人題署

HEALING WITH CHINESE HERBS

RICHARD HYATT

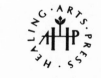

Healing Arts Press
Rochester, Vermont

Healing Arts Press
One Park Street
Rochester, Vermont 05767

Revised edition published 1990
First published in cloth by Schocken Books

Library of Congress Cataloging-in-Publication Data

Hyatt, Richard.
  Healing with Chinese herbs / Richard Hyatt.
    p.   cm.
  Includes bibliographical references.
  Rev. ed. of: Chinese herbal medicine.   1984, c1978.
  ISBN 0-89281-277-X
  1. Herbs—Therapeutic use. 2. Medicine, Chinese.   I. Hyatt,
Richard.   Chinese herbal medicine.   II. Title.
RM666.H33H94   1990
615. '321 '0951--dc20   90-30392
                                                                                CIP

Printed and bound in the United States

10 9 8 7 6 5 4 3

Healing Arts Press is a division of Inner Traditions International, Ltd.

Distributed to the book trade in Canada by Book Center, Inc.,
Montreal, Quebec

Distributed to the health food trade in Canada by Alive Books,
Toronto and Vancouver

The author wishes to impress upon the reader that this text is by no means to be considered a home medical adviser. If there is any truth in the proverb "A wise physician does not treat himself," then it must follow that a layman, even a wise layman, must seek out the aid of a qualified physician when in need. Some of these herbs can be extremely toxic when used incorrectly. In certain cases Chinese herbs alone would be insufficient to treat the illness and would be used in connection with acupuncture, diet, massage, and/or Western medicine. In such cases reliance on herbs alone could allow a disease to progress to a more serious stage. Chinese medicine is not a "folk" medicine but a highly developed art and science. Both intellectual acumen and practical experience are needed if its power is to be fully utilized.

CONTENTS

ACKNOWLEDGMENTS

It is customary to preface a work such as this with a few remarks acknowledging gratitude to those whose contributions and encouragement have helped to bring the material to the light of day. It is especially fitting here, where the author has served more as a scribe than a scholar, for there have been many without whom this work could not have begun and more still without whom it could never have been completed.

Whatever I may say will be inadequate to convey my initial indebtedness to Noburo Muramoto, the father of herbal medicine in America, for it was he who first had the courage to defy what was stagnant in an otherwise venerable tradition by teaching ear-whispered secrets to a Westerner. It was he who provided the original notes in Chinese upon which the section on herbal teas is based. I hope that by extending his work I have helped in some small measure to insure that my teacher's compassionate gesture and all the work it entailed for him were not undertaken in vain.

I am deeply indebted to my good friend and colleague Robert Feldman for his diligent and patient work in recovering invaluable research materials and for sharing these materials with me even before the publication of his own work.

I must also thank my teachers in other branches of the Oriental healing arts. Miss Shizuko Yamamoto deserves my thanks, for without her kindness and gentle guiding hand I might never have entered on this path. The many she has touched remain her legacy. I thank her for her patient tutelage in Shiatsu, the Japanese art of massage. In a like manner I must not fail to mention Michio Kushi and his wife, Aveline, who have done so much to further understanding of Oriental medicine, particularly in matters of diet and nutrition.

I must also thank my teachers in the martial arts for their many valuable criticisms and suggestions. In the traditional manner they are all masters of one or more healing arts. My Grand Master, Kuo Lien Ying, is a living example of the excellence of Chinese medicine. At age eighty-three he rises daily at 5:00 A.M. to practice Kung Fu. He has a ten-year-old son and can drink any of his students under the table. He is a Taoist of the first order and his medicine is the mastery of eternal youth.

10

To my wife, Chao Mei Kuei, I pledge my undying love and acknowledge here my thanks for her support in this work.

I wish to thank Mr. Leon Gubenow of the Downstate Medical Center Library for his help in finding difficult-to-locate manuscripts and for taking a personal interest in my work. I am indebted to Jim Chan and his daughter Fee for answering many questions pertaining to herbal formulae. I thank Naomi Wise, Chet Roaman, and especially Michael Goodwin for indispensable editorial direction. I am grateful to Jeffrey Michaels for assistance in difficult matters of Chinese translation. I should like to thank my good friend Mr. Shun Yu for lending his most talented hand to the rendering of the Chinese prescriptions included in this text. I am indebted to Professor Eugene Anderson of the University of California, Riverside, for his scholarly advice. I thank my typists, Mrs. Ruth Hyatt, Mr. Mo Kaplan, and Mr. Rudy Hohenstein. And to Annabelle Yen: thanks for being there when I needed you.

For whatever there is of value within these covers, praise is due entirely to my predecessors and teachers. For whatever is inadequate, misleading, or simply incorrect, I assume entire responsibility.

Richard Hyatt
Allhallows Eve, 1977
Berkeley, California

PREFACE

Ever since the Jesuit Friar Francis Xavier set foot in the Middle Kingdom, Western medicine has exerted a pervasive influence on the Orient without reciprocation. But now the introduction of acupuncture to the West has changed all that forever. Still, acupuncture is but one of many branches of Chinese medicine. The others await investigation.

Chinese herbal medicine is a healing art about which little is known in the West. Yet in China, where it has been practiced for thousands of years, herbal medicine has proven itself indispensable. Today on the mainland it is held in equal esteem with acupuncture and Western medicine.

Certainly an empirical medicine that has survived thousands of years of civilization has something to offer the West, if only in raw materials. Indeed, there is already evidence to substantiate that ground for investigation. Numerous modern drugs have their origins in Chinese medicine. A modern anticoagulant used to treat cerebral hemorrhage was first extracted from centrifuged leeches. The crude drug of dried leeches was prescribed for much the same purpose in Chinese medical texts eighteen hundred years ago. Ephedrine, a substance isolated from the crude drug Ma huang, is used in the treatment of asthma just as crude Ma huang has been traditionally used. Digitalis, perhaps the best-known wonder drug of Chinese origin, is an extract of Mao ti huang, another crude drug still used by Chinese physicians today as it has been for centuries. But these are merely examples of how Western medicine has used Chinese herbs to suit its own purposes. More recently there has been evidence in China to suggest that the crude drugs used in their unrefined state, according to the laws of traditional medicine, may often be more effective in treating certain diseases than our own modern variants. Like acupuncture, this evidence will in time become known to the world at large.

11

Up to now, unfortunately, little of this information has reached the general public, or even scientific circles, for that matter.

There have been many reasons for this, not the least of which is the linguistic problem. But even accounting for this formidable barrier, the material has been too long in coming to us. The primary obstacle preventing a systematic study of Oriental medicine until now has been a fundamental disparity between Oriental masters and prospective Western students in their approach to this study. As a rule the Westerner believes that an extensive theoretical study must precede any practical application of the material. The Oriental traditionalist, on the other hand, believes that theoretical investigation is only so much beating around the bush without the comparison of practical application. Thus the Western medical student devotes the early years of his education to rote memorization and theoretical dissertation, while the Oriental practitioner begins his first day's study at his master's elbow. As long as this basic disparity existed it was the prospective Western students who suffered, for the masters would have it their way.

Recently, though, a handful of forward-thinking Oriental masters, who recognized the need for change of the situation, have taken steps to remedy the matter. Numerous publications have been brought forth by students of these traditionalists, publications which have exposed previously unavailable knowledge in a form approachable by an audience with Western prejudices.

This step has been taken through the cooperation of the most recent generation of Oriental masters and their first generation of Western students. The young Westerners have won the confidence of their masters and an arrangement has been struck: the masters provide the information; the students dispense it through whatever form and vehicle they think will assure its revivification. This work is no exception.

The book has been arranged to provide a basic primer for the study of herbal medicine. The Introduction acquaints the reader with the history and traditions of Chinese herbal medicine. It is hoped that this history will instill the understanding that as a student of this path one enters into a tradition that is the legacy of individuals of high ideals and moral clarity. It is hoped that fledgling students will strive to measure up to their predecessors and carry on their good work for the sake of the alleviation of human suffering.

The theoretical section functions on two levels: for beginners it serves as an introduction to the principles of Oriental philosophy as they have traditionally applied to herbal medicine. Each of the subsections here (Yin and Yang, etc.) could by rights be a complete treatise in and of itself. However, as such a treatment is quite outside the scope of this work, these brief discussions must suffice. Of course most of the topics covered here are dealt with at length elsewhere, and the beginning student is expected to seek out such works and more thoroughly familiarize himself with these principles. (The bibliography provides direction in this.) For the intermediate or advanced student the theoretical section is designed to serve as a handbook-like distillation of basic principles. It will be useful because it provides the material essential to clinical practice in concise paragraphs and easy-to-use charts and graphs.

The Teas and Herbs sections are the heart of this text. This is the material that has previously been unavailable to anyone not fluent in written Chinese. Some of it has been published in translation in my teacher's book, *Healing Ourselves,* and in Masaru Toguchi's *Oriental Herbal Wisdom,* but these treatments are not complete and do not present the material in a form that facilitates practice. What has been lacking until now is a thorough cross-indexing of the romanized Chinese and Japanese names and their Latin counterparts as well as Chinese characters for these names. With the cross-indexing provided here a student can both develop the theoretical foundation of herbal medicine and obtain the materials necessary for its practice. The Chinese characters for the formulae enable a student to go to any of the herbal pharmacies listed in the appendix and present a prescription to be filled. Depending on the situation, a little sign language, pointing, and finger counting may be necessary, but the students who field tested this primer found that the Chinese characters and a little perseverance are all that are necessary to obtain the desired materials. Thus this text can be used in every stage of the study of herbal medicine, from general introduction to clinical practice. It should be understood that other written material may aid in this study and that the guidance of a qualified teacher should be sought and attained if possible. But acknowledging the limitations of our day and age, when these are unavailable, this text alone will suffice. This, and a measure of good judgment and correct purpose. We should recall the work and words of the barefoot doctors of China, who practice on themselves to develop the skill necessary to treat the rural masses. They say, "To practice medicine we must practice fearless materialism," and, "It would be better to harm ourselves than to harm a single hair on the head of one of the people." This is the correct attitude.

The purpose of this book is to provide for the first time in English a substantial exposition of Chinese herbal medicine, as well as a detailed presentation of many of the formulae and crude drugs that comprise the Chinese pharmacopeia. Having developed out of the largest, most populous, and longest-enduring civilization in the world, the sources and variety of Chinese herbs are almost beyond categorical analysis.

This work cannot constitute a complete catalogue of Chinese herbal medicine. Nor can it hope to serve as a thorough compendium of the principles of diagnosis, pathology, and clinical technique. What it can hope to accomplish is to introduce the practice of herbal medicine to the West and to bring to light the work of many dedicated scholars both East and West who foresaw the potential of this study for serving humanity.

CHINESE HERBAL MEDICINE

An Ancient Art and Modern Healing Science

Chapter 1
INTRODUCTION:
The History of
Chinese Herbal
Medicine

The West adheres to the notion of linear, chronological development with one event following another in ordered sequence, the earlier events generating and influencing later ones in more or less equal proportion to their proximity. The Chinese, on the other hand, have traditionally viewed history as a series of temporal cycles, each distinctly separated from the others, the largest of these being the great religious epochs and political dynasties. We might say that the Westerner tends to view his age in history as one in a series of blocks lined up each in front of the other, whereas the traditional Chinese has tended to view his age as a sphere in a planetarium, where each sphere exists separate from the others while retaining a similar proximity to all. The significant thing about the Chinese concept is that it allows a far-distant planet by virtue of its brilliance to cast a more pervasive influence on our own orb than might another closer but less radiant body. This perspective has led to a timeless atmosphere in which relatively little differentiation need be made between the most recent theories and techniques and those of centuries ago. Consequently the Chinese approach has been to place emphasis, not on progress in technology, but on sorting, refining, and evaluating what has been known and practiced in the past, and on applying this information along with new knowledge to the formulation of a wholistic cosmology that is appropriate for the present. Always the direction has been to stress development in the field of dialectics and theory while keeping technique refined, generalized, and simplified.

Chinese medicine has always been a medicine of empiricism. Those concepts that have come to us from remote eras have endured not merely out of deference to the ancient but because they have proven themselves sound in centuries of practice.

The origin of Chinese medicine is usually associated with three legendary emperors: Fu Hsi, Shen Nung, and Huang Ti.

Fu Hsi's reign began in 2852 B.C. He is credited with the most profound accomplishment in Chinese history, the formulation of the yin yang doctrine. It is the cornerstone of Chinese philosophy. As this doctrine is the basis of the *I Ching* or *Book of Changes,* the oldest of all Chinese books, Fu Hsi is credited with its authorship. Several translations of the text are available in English, the best of these being the Wilhelm/Baynes translation (see Bibliography).

Shen Nung, the second of these emperors, is the father of agriculture and herbal medicine. He is thought to have invented the plow and is given credit for authorship of the first native herbal, the *Shen Nung Pen Ts'ao*, translated simply as *Shen Nung's Herbal,* on the basis of his own experimentation. According to popular legend every day he would go out into the fields, marshes, and forests and conduct research on the native botanicals, eating them whenever necessary. It is said that he poisoned himself eighty times a day, but since he was a great physician he always recovered. Even today he is held in esteem as the patron saint of herbalism. His reign ended in the year 2697 B.C.

The third emperor, Huang Ti, reigned from 2697 to 2595 B.C. He was the first true emperor, as it was he who established court, rank, and ritual. The most prolific of the three sovereigns, he is known as the inventor of the first wheeled vehicle, the chariot. His other important inventions include ships, the planetarium, cloth clothing, currency, and musical notation, among numerous others. He is also credited with authorship of the *Huang Ti Nei Ching,* translated as *The Yellow Emperor's*

Classic of Internal Medicine, the most important and earliest extant work on Chinese medicine (see Bibliography).

According to Eugene Anderson, Professor of Anthropology at the University of California, Riverside, "No serious scholar questions the mythological nature of the three emperors. Fu Hsi is said to have had the body of a giant snake; Shen Nung simply means divine farmer; and The Yellow Emperor is equally improbable."

The *Shen Nung Pen Ts'ao* was actually written in the Han dynasty (206 B.C.–220 A.D.), and the earliest fragments of the *Nei Ching* date back only a few centuries B.C. Doubtless these works were fathered on their illustrious namesakes in the hope that it would help to enhance their authority.

According to another popular legend, around the year 1500 B.C. a cook in the emperor's kitchen named I-Yin served the court a decoction of several different herbs. The people of the court enjoyed the taste, but, more important, many of them recognized its beneficial medicinal effect. The idea caught on and soon became the most common means of administering crude drugs. Thus I-Yin was established as the originator of herb teas or soups (t'ang).

The earliest medical references are to be found in the *Tso Chuan,* a history carved in stone at Loyang around 240 A.D. and possibly dating as early as 540 B.C. This does not, however, signify the beginnings of Chinese medicine, merely the beginning of its recorded history. It seems likely that Chinese medicine was of a much earlier origin and was probably transmitted by oral tradition and etchings on bone.

India was the first foreign civilization to have an effect in shaping indigenous Chinese medicine. The golden age of Buddhism in India was a time that saw much of India's culture, including Ayurvedic medicine, carried abroad by continental and maritime expansion. Early in the era Ayurvedic medicine reached China, where it was readily assimilated.

At about this time Tsou Yen (c. 305–240 B.C.), who probably had some contact with Indian travelers, tried to amalgamate Chinese medical dialectics with the philosophy of Indian Ayurvedic medicine. In doing so he developed the wu hsing, or five-element theory, after which Chinese medicine was constructed upon a system of elements and vital spirits, like its Indian and Greek counterparts. As the similarities suggest, it is entirely possible that the theory of the elements originally came from Greece, was transmitted through India, and finally reached China from there.

Medical theory was not the only importation to influence China at this time. Other, more concrete barters were received as well. For example, of the 779 herbs in the *Pen Ts'ao (Native Herbal)*, all are from India, and more than fifty are of Arab-Iranian origin.

Contemporary with the Roman Empire, the Han dynasty represents the emergence of China as a world power. By this time China had direct or indirect contact with the Middle East, India, Southeast Asia, and the Mediterranean via maritime and overland trade routes. The economy and culture were stable, and this stimulated all forms of scientific development, medicine included. Through the *Han Shu (Annals of the Han)* we know that four important medical works were circulated at the time: the *I Ching (Classic of Medicine)*, the *Ching Fang (Collection of Prescriptions)*, the *Fang Chung (Treatise on Sex and Hygiene)*, and the *Shen Hsien (Methods and Prescriptions for Attaining Immortality)*. Unfortunately, all these works are lost. The only book from Han times available to us today is the *Nei Ching (Classic of Internal Medicine)*. Under the Han dynasty the classical doctrine of Chinese medicine was formulated. The great masters of the period were Chang Chung Ching and Hua To.

Chang Chung Ching (born c. 158–166) is known as the Chinese Hippocrates. He was the first codifier of Chinese symptomology and therapeutics. He was also the first to systematically differentiate clearly between yin and yang symptoms. His major accomplishment for posterity is the authorship of the *Shang Han Lun (Treatise on Ailments Attributed to the Cold)*, a text every bit as important as the *Nei Ching*. This treatise describes the development of diseases caused by the cold as occurring in stages and identifies these according to their symptoms. Herbal decoctions are then prescribed for treatment of the various stages. Even today this text is the bedside handbook of the young traditional physician. Despite its importance it remains the only one of the basic classics not yet translated into English.

Hua To (born c. 136–141) was the outstanding surgeon of this period. Aside from his work as a surgeon—he was the inventor of sutures—he was also an acupuncturist, an anatomist, and a physical therapist. He is thought to have published (under a pseudonym) charts showing the arrangement of the organs inside the body. Hua To was very much interested in the study of drugs. He was the first to use anesthetics, antiseptics, anti-inflammatory ointments, and anthelmintics. As a physical therapist he originated the use of medicinal baths along with hydrotherapy. He also observed that physical culture facilitated digestion and circulation and strengthened the body. On the basis of these observations he originated the five animal exercises, modeled after the movements of the tiger, stag, bear, monkey, and crane. This series of exercises is thought to have greatly influenced the Chinese martial arts as we know them today. Before Hua To's influence was felt, the martial arts were probably primarily concerned with flailing techniques, with little emphasis on breath control and anatomy. During his later life, Hua To fell into disfavor with the emperor and perished as a result. He never published his own works, though while in prison he composed works intended for publication. The text that bears his name today, *Hua Shih Chung Tsang Ching,* is only an apocryphal compilation written quite recently by Sun Sing Yen (1753–1818).

The era of the Taoists spans several dynasties reaching from the third century B.C. to the seventh century A.D. From the very inception of indigenous medicine, through the formative years and right up into the golden age of the Tang dynasty, Taoist yogis, hygienists, and philosophers were involved every step of the way. During the third to sixth century A.D. the Taoists rose to their greatest prominence.

Ko Hung (281–340) was one of the great Taoist doctors. Unlike most of the scholars of his age, he was not blessed with a wealthy family to finance his education. As a youth he worked as a laborer to support his studies. Having little inclination for leisure, he readily gave himself over to the study of ancient texts and the practice of breathing exercises. Writing under the pseudonym Pao Pu Tzu, he composed two important medical texts as well as a treatise on esoteric Taoist practices. His medical texts are *Chin Kuei Yo Fang (Medications from the Golden Box)* and *Chou-Hou Pei-Tsi Fang (First Aid Measures)*, later completed by T'ao as *The Hermit's Book of 100 Recipes*.

Ko Hung was gravely concerned with the need for putting inexpensive, readily available medicines within the reach of everyone. To this end he devoted eight chapters of *Chou-Hou Pei-Tsi Fang* to the subject "Prescriptions Ready to Hand."

T'ao Hung Ching (452–536) was another master Taoist. Influenced by Buddhism as well as Taoism, he was a Renaissance man: mathematician, astronomer, calligrapher, pharmacologist, and physician. From an early age he devoted himself wholeheartedly to the study of all kinds of books. He was particularly influenced by his predecessor, Ko Hung. He served in the imperial court for a while, but in later life relinquished wealth and position to lead the life of a mountain hermit and continue his research. T'ao composed and edited an annotated version of the *Shen Nung Pen Ts'ao,* part of which was recovered at the caves of Tun-huang toward the end of the Ming dynasty. Though some of the material in T'ao's *Pen Ts'ao* is very old, the greater part was composed by an unknown writer of the early Han whose sources did not go beyond the fourth century B.C.

Some time after the decline of the Han dynasty a reunification of Chinese territories took place under the Sui and Tang dynasties (590–618 and 618–906 respectively). From 618 to 741 the stability of the political situation encouraged rapid development of the national culture and economy. Many noteworthy achievements were made in the field of medicine. The science was reorganized completely, and its study was approved by examinations under the control of the T'ai i shu (Grand Medical Service), formed in 624. It is one of the earliest examples of the teaching of medicine under state control. This was the golden age of the Tang dynasty, the era when Chinese medicine reached its zenith.

Sun Szu Miao (581–682) was outstanding among the monk doctors of the period, a splendid example of the selfless men

who were involved in the study of medicine. The son of a scholar, he began his study of Taoist texts and the Buddhist canons at
the age of seven. Early in life he withdrew to the Tapo Moun-
tains to live as a hermit, but his renown was such that two
emperors, Emperor Wen of the Sui dynasty and Emperor Kao
Tsung of the Tang, summoned him to court with offers of high
position. He declined on the pretext of illness and remained at
his hermitage in the tradition of the great Chinese sages. He died
at the advanced age of a hundred and one. Throughout his life he
wrote extensively; his works on herbal medicine are known as
Ts'ien Chin Fang (1000 Precious Recipes) and *Ts'ien Chin I (Supplement to 1000 Precious Recipes)*.

It was during the Tang dynasty that the *Nei Ching* took the
form in which it has come down to us today. The work's earliest
fragments date back to the third to fifth century B.C., at which
time it must have been a homogeneous composition. During the
Ch'in period (221–206 B.C.) it seems to have been divided into
two parts. The Su Wen, which is composed of nine chapters and
is mainly theoretical, and the Ling Shu, which is also nine chapters and is primarily practical. A great deal of material appears to
have been added after this division, as all passages alluding to
the six hollow organs are known to be more recent than the first
century of the Christian era. During the sixth century, under the
Sui dynasty, the Su Wen was known to consist of only eight of
the original nine scrolls. Under the Tang, two more scrolls, the
seventh and ninth, were also lost. Thus this text, which so many
scholars have regarded as very ancient, must in light of ar-
cheological evidence be considered a composite work constantly
modified from the earliest eras to the Tang dynasty, when its
form was finally fixed.

In the period 742–820 corruption set in and the recurrence of
civil war weakened China. From 821 onward the rise to power of
the eunuchs signaled the decline of the Tang.

After the fall of the Tang dynasty, the Northern Sung dynasty
(960–1126) was never able to achieve a reunification of Chinese
territories. But the political and military defeats of the age were
offset by great accomplishments in the arts and sciences. It was
during the Sung period that Chan (or Zen) or Buddhism rose to

predominance and greatly influenced the arts. This age saw the invention of the compass, printing, and gunpowder. In medicine new developments included forensic medicine, protective vario- lation, and the casting of bronze acupuncture mannequins to facilitate teaching. The materia medica was expanded in con- junction with progress in zoology and botany, and the new em- phasis on trade and cultural exchange with southern neighbors. Among the new crude drugs to enter the Chinese pharmacopeia at this time were mandragora, myrrh, theriac, fenugreek, and opium. For the first time collections of articles on medicine began to be compiled and republished in encyclopedias printed from wood blocks and sometimes illustrated in color.

During the Sung dynasty, Chen Si I edited a text compiled by Yuan Liou Chuang (also known as Chung Chih). After its republi- cation somewhat later, during the Ch'ing dynasty, it became the classic on the subject of physiognomy. Its title is *Shen Sang Ts'uan Pien (Complete Treatise on the Connection Between the Mind and the External Features of the Body)*. According to this work, by careful observation of a patient's features a diagnosti- cian can deduce that individual's character traits, clinical condi- tion, and probable future. As organic failures often produce changes in the features, this system does have some scientific basis. Over the years it has proven itself very useful.

The Yuan dynasty (1279–1368) found China dominated by the Mongol legions of the Khans. Devastation and destruction were visited upon the nation, and its culture suffered immensely. There were serious famines and pestilence. The population de- creased from one hundred million (c. 1125) to sixty million (c. 1290). No significant advances were made in the field of medicine. Ironically, China's boundaries reached their greatest expansion at this time.

Thrust into power by a peasant revolt, the Ming dynasty (1368–1644) ended the Mongol rule of China. It freed Peking, which had been in the hands of the Mongols for 432 years; and a capital was established there. The new dynasty was anxious to reestablish the intellectual and moral values of old China, and a spectacular, albeit short-lived, neoclassical period ensued. However, under the burden of so long a Mongolian rule, much of the fabric of Chinese culture had worn thin. Within a relatively short time the cultural resources were exhausted, and in over-zealous attempts to mimic the Tang, stagnation set in within all the arts and sciences. The decline of the Ming began after the reign of Yung Lo (1403–1424).

The arrival of the Jesuits in Peking in 1601 would have exposed China to Western science and medicine had this not been stopped short by Emperor Kang Hsi, who considered these ideas too revolutionary. Fearing that they might disturb the harmony of Chinese civilization, he chose to suppress their circulation among the people and instead kept the Jesuits and their curious knowledge for his own amusement.

In the latter days of the Ming dynasty, Li Shih Chen (1518–1593) composed his materia medica, the *Pen Ts'ao Kang Mu*. It is the pièce de résistance of the modern age of traditional medicine, perhaps the only important original work to follow the age of Mongol rule. It ranks with the *Nei Ching* and *Shang Han Lun* as one of the three most important books on Chinese medicine. Aside from its unsurpassed value as a catalogue of pathology and therapeutics, it is also a source book of natural science, giving classifications of mineral, vegetable, and animal products, as well as accounts of technological, geographical, dietetic, culinary, cosmological, philosophical, and philological information.

The Ch'ing dynasty (1644–1911) was again a dynasty of foreign domination. The Manchus ruled China for 250 years and were able, in their time, to repeat the Mongols' bid for universal power. However, they never succeeded in being assimilated by the Chinese people. They suffered constant harrassment from Ming legitimists, nonconformist scholars, secret revolutionary societies, peasant and minority uprisings, and piracy on the high seas. Moreover, conservative, feudalistic northern China, with its center in Peking, was being overtaken by maritime, commercial southern China, centered in Canton and already open to Western influence.

This was the time when Protestant missionaries brought Western medicine to supplant the traditional practices. This might not have occurred had not the system of Chinese medicine already fallen into decay due to elitism. The official medicine served only the court. Its practitioners were schooled in such dubious accomplishments as the careful drafting of unbesmudged prescriptions and the composition of essays that relied heavily on quotations from the classics. The system was a feeble re-creation of its Tang predecessor and failed miserably insofar as the training of competent physicians was concerned, especially any capable of serving the needs of the people. The common citizenry was reduced to dependence on street-corner healers who ranged from soothsayers to barber-masseurs. Although the outstanding doctors of earlier times had gone to great pains to distinguish themselves from sorcerers, they had never completely succeeded in dissociating classical medicine from magic in the minds of the masses. Now, in the declining days of the Chinese empire, the tendency to link the two became rampant. Eventually the rational classical approach lost appeal for common citizenry and ruling aristocracy alike, and they turned to the occult in its stead. This movement was stimulated by certain deviant forms of Buddhism and Taoism, and by the resurgence of local shamanism. As charms, prayers, exorcisms, talismans, and potions became increasingly popular, the shamans and priests made a nice livelihood providing them.

The Boxer Rebellion marked the end of the dark age of magic and superstition. It was succeeded by an era of growing concern for immediate social and national needs. New China was emerging.

At the turn of the century traditional medicine still held an important place among the people, but it began to lose favor among the cultivated elite, many of whom had studied or traveled abroad. The court medical college was at its nadir. Teaching had come to a standstill and the care of the imperial family comprised the sole activity of its members. Schools teaching traditional medicine were closed one after another. Their complete closure was envisioned for 1929. During the period of the Republic (1912–1949), only eight still functioned.

But no matter how significant the modernist movement was, it could not persuade millions of peasants to give up their native medicine. Nor could it close down the centuries old crude-drug industry that provided a livelihood for so many people. For one thing, this medicine was familiar to the people. Western medicine was not. More significant, the average person simply did not have access to Western medicine, even if he would have chosen it. So instead of disappearing, traditional medicine simply went underground. This was an important period of evolution, for it was a time when traditional medicine lost many of the useless frills it had acquired, while the tried-and-true techniques endured. Though traditional medicine was dormant, it nevertheless still possessed considerable potency. And it went on to prove its usefulness.

During the many years of fighting against the Japanese and Republican forces, the leaders of the emerging People's Republic of China could not help noticing that this medicine was of indispensable service to the troops. It was better suited to the situation and the environment than Western medicine, which relied heavily on highly refined supplies not easy to come by in China's vast rural expanses. Thus Chinese medicine proved itself after all to be neither feudal nor reactionary, but indeed a medicine of the people. This is not surprising, for in its finest hours it had always been. In view of this, traditional medicine was restored to official esteem after liberation in 1949.

Since then, specialist hospitals have been set up in Peking, Tientsin, Shanghai, Nanking, Chungking, Wuhan, Sian, Harbin, Kunming, Nanchang, and elsewhere. So have twenty universities of traditional medicine, chairs on the history of traditional medicine, a journal, a pharmacological laboratory, an Academy of Acupuncture, and a Central Research Institute of Traditional Medicine. In 1954 traditional doctors and Western doctors were brought together in the Chinese Medical Association to see if the two groups could make a united effort based on mutual understanding. This brought about a drastic change in the mentality of some half a million traditional doctors schooled in the ancient fashion, as their system was exposed to the harsh light of scientific method. But it was no more severe than the shock received by modern doctors when the traditionalists went on to meet the challenge and produced results which the scientists found difficult to explain. The significant thing is that the two groups were able to see eye to eye on such basic issues as priorities and the development of a common front against disease from a synthesis of two lines of thought as different as yin and yang. Today modern doctors and traditionalists work together in hospitals throughout China.

A broad plan for the future of Chinese medicine has been outlined and its initial stages are already in effect. The first step is to align with Western medicine in the prevention of disease; the second, to integrate with modern medicine and extend that integration to encompass all medical activity among the people; and the third, to make available all that is of value from traditional medicine for assimilation by world science.

While the obstacles raised in bringing together two such dissimilar doctrines are clearly formidable, they are not insurmountable. The integration of traditional and Western medicine will no doubt be a long and arduous undertaking, but it is of the greatest importance to both China and the world. The future of traditional medicine looks promising.

Chapter 2
THEORY AND FUNDAMENTAL PRINCIPLES

A Chinese proverb says, "Nature cures the disease, the doctor collects the fee." The basic idea of this statement is correct, but in truth the proverb falls somewhat short of the mark. When a physician has reached the highest level of judgment, his mind is empty of preconceptions. At such a level his medicine takes on an almost spiritual aura.

The great sages sought to master all fields of human endeavor necessary for self-sufficiency. Holding to this ideal, educated individuals in the Far East have traditionally studied martial arts for self-protection, medicine for self-preservation, and the fine arts and literature for self-expression. Because of the wide scope and integration of this study, Oriental philosophy developed with a breadth and integrity that allows for its application to every one of these fields. By the same token these separate fields of study developed with profound simplicity and with a generalizing approach to technique that would not necessitate overspecialization.

To a person unacquainted with Oriental culture the principles of Oriental medicine may seem vague, archaic, superstitious. However, upon further study Oriental philosophy will be found to embody deep wisdom expressed through a highly refined yet fundamentally simple dialectic. The various theories of Oriental medicine merely serve to relate the diversified information necessary for the application of abstract dialectic principles to practical technique.

Oriental medicine is composed of three inseparable parts: technique, theory, and sensitivity. Of the three, sensitivity is the most important. Technique is the easiest to learn. Theory is the bridge between the two. Almost every peasant mother knows something of technique. But only those who devote much time and energy to the study of theory ever develop the intuition necessary to employ this technique to the fullest.

It is appropriate here to state emphatically that theory will become clear only through practice. Traditionally such practice is performed under the guidance of a qualified master, or, when one is lacking, with the greatest caution on oneself. Conceptual knowledge will never substitute for practical experience.

Yin and Yang

"The Yin Yang principle is the basic principle of the entire universe. It is the principle of everything in creation. It brings about all change; it is the root source of Life and Death, it is found within the temples of the Gods.

"In order to treat and cure diseases, one must search into their origins. Heaven was created by an accumulation of Yang 陽 , the light element, while earth was created by an accumulation of Yin 陰 , the dark element. Through their interactions and functions, Yin and Yang, the negative and positive principle in nature, are responsible for the diseases which befall those who are in rebellion against the laws of nature."

So says the *Nei Ching, The Yellow Emperor's Classic of Internal Medicine*.

The doctrine of yin yang is the fundamental principle employed by all classical Chinese arts and sciences. The oldest written reference to the principle occurs in the Chou Government's *Book of Rites,* dated as eleventh century B.C. Its origin is credited to Fu Hsi, the first of China's legendary emperors.

The old hieroglyphic character for yang is a picture of the sun with its rays emanating, combined with a picture of a mountain. The image is "the sunny side of a mountain." The old character for yin shows a picture of a cloud with one of a mountain. The image is "the dark side of a mountain." Each is opposite to the other in nature, yet they both hold the mountain in common. They are complementary in that the existence of one implies that of the other.

Today, writes Stephan Palos, the official view of the People's Republic of China is that the yin yang principle "contains an original, spontaneously dialectical, and simple materialist doctrine; it is free of superstition; it approximates scientific formulation; and it represents a progressive way of thinking."

Yin and yang are idealized states. In reality neither exists in absolute, only in relativity to the other. (What is yang in one situation may be yin in another.) These conditions are mutually complementary and antagonistic. Yang is the positive active state, characterized by heat, light, and the exterior. Its gender is male. Yin is the negative inactive state, more precisely the absence of yang, characterized by cold, darkness, and the interior. Its gender is female. Neither exist as a static condition, for both are in a perpetual state of transformation, continually blending with each other in greater or lesser proportions. There is always some yin in yang and some yang in yin. People are subject to and reflect the cyclic variations of this principle. They are more active during the day and in summer, more passive during the night and the winter. The organs, too, follow the variations of this change. Thus illness or malfunction of the organs can be addressed as merely an abnormal accumulation of yin or yang, a temporary condition that can be transformed by compliance with the natural activity of yin and yang.

The healthy body is constantly changing from yin to yang and from yang to yin. The physician encourages this change but avoids extremes. If at any time the body condition diverts from this orderly course and becomes increasingly yin or yang, disease arises. This simple concept is the fundamental theory for prescribing herbal medicine. For example, yang herbs such as jen shen or fu tzu, which are tonics or hypertensives, are used for persons suffering from yin conditions such as low blood pressure or general debility. Yin herbs such as ta huang (a laxative and hypotensive) are used for persons suffering from yang conditions such as high blood pressure or chronic constipation. Every herb has its particular yin yang character. When herbs are used in combination infinite variations are possible; an appropriate herbal remedy can be formulated for any possible condition of disease.

Thus the application of yin yang to Oriental medical treatment is very simple and straightforward. Once the physician has explained the laws governing yin yang to his patient, the patient is encouraged to comply with them.

Qualities of Yin Yang

	YIN	YANG
Tendency	To Condense	To Develop
Position	Inward	Outward
Structure	Space	Time
Direction	Descending (to earth)	Rising (to heaven)
Color	Purple	Red
Temperature	Cold	Hot
Weight	Heavy	Light
Catalyst	Water	Fire
Light	Dark	Bright
Construction	Interior	Exterior (surface)
Work	Psychological	Physical
Attitude	Gentle, Negative	Active, Positive
Biological Classification	Vegetable	Animal
Sex	Female	Male
Nerves	Orthosympathetic	Parasympathetic
Taste	Hot, Sour	Sweet, Bitter
Seasonal Correspondence	Winter	Summer

LAWS GOVERNING YIN YANG

Axioms

1. All things are the differentiated apparatus of one infinity.
2. Everything changes.
3. All antagonisms are complementary.
4. No two things are identical.

5. Every condition has its opposite.
6. The extremity of any condition is equal in its opposite.
7. Whatever has a beginning has an end.

Theorems

1. Infinity divides itself into yin and yang.
2. Yin and yang result continuously from the infinite movement of the universe.
3. Yin is centripetal. Yang is centrifugal. Together they produce all energy and phenomena.
4. Yin attracts yang. Yang attracts yin.
5. Yin repels yin. Yang repels yang.
6. The force of attraction and repulsion between any two things is proportional to the difference in their yin yang constitution.
7. All phenomena are ephemeral and constantly changing their yin yang constitution.
8. Nothing is solely yin or yang; everything involves polarity.
9. Nothing is neuter. Either yin or yang is always in excess.
10. Yin and yang are relative. Large yin attracts small yin. Large yang attracts small yang.
11. At the extremity of their manifestation, yin produces yang and yang produces yin.
12. All physical forms are yin at the center and yang at the surface.

Further Differentiations of Yin and Yang

To adapt the yin yang theory to more precise application, it is necessary to further differentiate yin and yang into four categories: old yang, young yang, young yin, and old yin. These categories represent progressive stages in a process of change from extreme yang to extreme yin. (It is important to remember that extreme yang does not mean absolute yang and vice versa. Nothing in existence is solely yin or yang. Thus the four categories represent degrees of dominance of yin and yang.)

To complicate matters, traditional Chinese practitioners use three sets of terminology to note these categories. We have already used one set (old yang, young yang, young yin, old yin), but there are two more. They are: (1) big yang, small yang, small yin, big yin; and (2) full yang, empty yang, full yin, empty yin. Generally speaking, the terms "young" and "old" are employed for pure theory, "big" and "small" for applied theory, and "full" and "empty" for medical practice. However, for most practical purposes they are interchangeable.

The following table may be helpful:

old yang	young yang	young yin	old yin
big yang	small yang	small yin	big yin
full yang	empty yang	full yin	empty yin

It should be noted that the third set of terms (full yang, empty yang, full yin, empty yin) does not seem to exhibit the mirror symmetry of the first two sets. The reason for this is simple (though a bit confusing at first). "Big," "old," "young," and "small" modify yin and yang as more or less extreme, while "full" and "empty" modify them as more or less yin or yang, "full" meaning yangness and "empty" meaning yinness. When in doubt, a glance at the table above may be helpful.

This differentiation may be illustrated through use of the yin yang symbols of the *I Ching*. If a solid line represents yang and a broken line yin, the four differentiations can be illustrated by doubling the lines:

old yang	young yang	young yin	old yin
————	—— ——	————	—— ——
————	————	—— ——	—— ——

Each of these configurations has its own distinct yin yang value. Understanding the difference between the extreme polarities (i.e., old yang and old yin) is fairly simple. But understanding the difference between young yang and young yin requires more careful consideration. One unfamiliar with the laws governing yin yang might conclude that the two configurations are neuter and equal. This *is not* the case. (Remember Theorem 9.) Again, an illustration will help to clarify this.

In building the images used in the *I Ching,* one begins with a base line and adds lines toward the top. Thus the original yang line configuration gives rise to two double line configurations, each having a solid line base:

The same is true of the yin image:

Though both young images contain one yin line and one yang line, they differ in that one is formed by adding a yin line to an already established lower yang line, while the other is formed by adding a yang line to an already established lower yin line. It is the lower (or "foundation") line that decides whether the image is yin or yang.

In applying this theory to medical practice, the patient's physical constitution may be considered the lower (or "foundation") line. That is, any individual will be either yin or yang, a base state (determined by such factors as bone structure, etc.) that will change very little during a lifetime. The factors that correspond to the upper line (and determine whether the patient's condition is old or young within the base state) are more easily changed factors, such as hyper- or hypoactivity of body organs.

Although it is easy to tell the difference between an old yang and old yin condition, the difference between a small yang and small yin condition may be subtle but its observance is just as important. A serious error can be made in judging a small yang situation as small yin. For example, while thinking one is encouraging the attraction of yin to yang (as noted in Theorem 4), one might mistakenly be encouraging the attraction of small yang for greater yang (as noted in Theorem 10), thus worsening an already yang situation. In applying theory one tries always to maintain a condition of balance (or, more accurately, a dynamic equilibrium of oscillation) between yin and yang. Extremes of yin and yang must be avoided.

BIG AND SMALL YIN AND YANG

Once a careful judgment has been made, one should encourage change to the opposite "young" condition, regardless of whether the existing condition is a young or an old one. For instance, if one is fortunate and finds himself faced with a young yin or young yang situation, he should encourage change to its young opposite, yang or yin respectively. If, on the other hand, one encounters a situation that has reached an extreme, he should encourage change not to the opposite extreme, but rather to the opposite young condition.

Three examples of harmonious change:

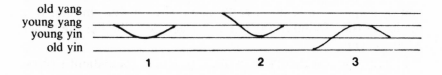

An example of undisciplined change:

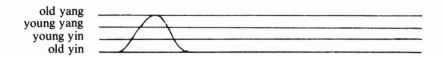

This concept of seeking balanced conditions while avoiding extremes is one of the most fundamental rules governing the practical application of yin yang theory. It is employed for both diagnosis and treatment in herbal medicine as well as the other branches of Oriental medicine. It is also central to all the traditional Chinese arts and sciences. It must be clearly understood before thorough study of these is possible.

Empty Full

The empty full theory categorizes body types into four generalized groups, full yang, empty yang, full yin, and empty yin, each corresponding to a division of the young and old yin yang principle. Remedial action is then prescribed for treatment of the chronic diseases that often afflict people of each body type. Traditionally, certain herb teas are employed to achieve the desired actions.

Full yang people tend to be active, to have reddish complexions, and to be overweight. They generally suffer from high blood pressure and overactive organs. They are likely to develop heart trouble and may develop cerebral hemorrhage or tuberculosis. Treatment prescribes herb teas to induce vomiting and diarrhea. Traditionally, chu chu'ueh t'ang (Japanese, sugyakuto) is listed as the specific herbal tea, but this is a very strong tea and for that reason it has been used much less in recent years. Often it may be wisely replaced by one of the cheng chi teas, which do not induce vomiting and are less likely to produce harmful side effects.

Empty yang people are those who are active, have brownish or tan complexions, and are thin but muscular. They are generally healthy but they are prone to develop kidney diseases. Treatment suggests making the person warm.

Full yin people are those who are not very active, have a yellowish tinge to the complexion, and have a tendency to become overweight. Such people are prone to develop liver diseases. Traditional treatment is to bring about sweating.

Empty yin people are those who are inactive, have pale complexions, are thin, and generally lack energy and vitality. They usually suffer from anemia and are likely to develop lung trouble and tuberculosis.

The following table gives the herbal teas traditionally used to produce the effects required for treatment of these conditions.

BODY TYPE	SYMPTOMS	TREATMENT
full yang	active red complexion overweight	Induce discharge: Hsiao ch'eng ch'i t'ang
empty yang	active tan thin and muscular	Make warm: Chen wu t'ang Szu ni t'ang Wu wei keng t'ang
full yin	somewhat inactive yellowish complexion somewhat overweight	Induce sweating: Ma huang t'ang Hsiao ch'ing lung t'ang
empty yin	inactive pale underweight	Induce harmony: Pai hu chia jen shen t'ang Li chung t'ang Fu tzu t'ang Szu ni t'ang

In conjunction with the empty full theory, Oriental medicine uses a system for the classification and treatment of chronic diseases that affect any of the three important humors: water, blood, and chi. It is employed in cases in which a disease has progressed beyond the general empty full condition and has condensed into symptoms of a specified order. Oriental medicine does not usually place significance on the localization of disease, as such emphasis might suggest treatment for the removal of local symptoms rather than treatment for overall improvement of the whole being. Although this method of treatment is somewhat symptomatic (in that it classifies diseases as belonging to one humor or another, and focuses treatment accordingly), it is still a general theory in that treatment has an overall curative effect on the humor under treatment, and indirectly on the whole body.

The water disease category includes all diseases associated with retention of water, and the urinary and excretory systems. The most prominent symptom of water disease is swelling. Other symptoms are unusual urination or bowel movements, or sweating. Of the three types, this category of disease is thought to be the easiest to cure; improvement is generally swift once the treatment is begun.

Blood disease includes all conditions associated with malfunctions of the circulatory system. This covers blood stagnation, anemia, varicose veins, hardening of arteries, hemorrhage, and so on. These diseases are more severe than water diseases, but they too can be treated effectively. Improvement is generally perceivable soon after treatment is begun, except in stubborn cases when the condition has prevailed for a very long time. In such cases considerable time may elapse before the patient begins to improve, though frequently the improvement will continue and gain in momentum once it has begun.

Chi may be defined as the "life force," equivalent to prana in the Sanskrit terminology. It is the subtle energy that permeates all living beings and is found in great concentration along the acupuncture meridians. Chi disease is the category most dreaded by Oriental physicians, for this category encompasses the most elusive diseases known to man. Chi diseases are those affecting the nervous system, the acupuncture meridian system, and the mind. Such diverse conditions as schizophrenia and Parkinson's disease are included in this category.

The origins of chi diseases are very hard to diagnose. People with no symptoms of serious imbalance whatever may suffer from these diseases, along with those who display symptoms of every type of degenerative condition. Even when diagnosed, treatment is often next to impossible. Oriental medicine leaves the ultimate responsibility for the cure with the patient himself. In cases of chi disease a patient often cannot or will not collaborate with nature and the doctor. Therefore the greatest tact and good judgment is necessary in dealing with patients suffering from chi diseases. Even great masters have failed to completely cure such diseases. Rarely will a patient respond to treatment immediately. More often he will improve only after extensive treatment. In other cases a patient may respond well for a while and then fail to improve further, or even revert to his original condition. There is no general rule for recovery from chi diseases. This is the primary reason they are so difficult to treat.

The following table lists the teas most commonly used in treating water, blood, and chi diseases.

Symptoms and Teas

DISEASE AND SYMPTOMS	BODY TYPE	TEA
water disease:	yang full	W'u ling t'ang
swelling	yang empty	Pa wei wan
	yin full	Wu ling t'ang
	yin empty	Chen wu t'ang
blood disease:	yang full	Ts'ao ho ch'eng ch'i t'ang
blood stagnation	yang empty	T'ang kuei t'iao yao san
	yin full	Kuei chih fu ling wan
	yin empty	Li chung t'ang
		Szu chun tzu t'ang
chi disease:	yang full	Ta ch'eng ch'i t'ang
nervous and mental	yang empty	Pan hsia hou pu t'ang
disorders	yin full	Ch'ai hu chia lung ku mu li t'ang
	yin empty	Kuei chih chia lung ku mu li t'ang

Stages of Disease

Diseases are dynamic conditions. Over the course of their development they change drastically with regard to the symptoms they manifest. Accordingly, treatment must be modified to suit the various stages of development of a disease.

Classifying different stages in the development of diseases in conjunction with the different body conditions is one of the greatest innovations of Oriental medicine. Under this system the two factors are weighed together to reach an individual and timely diagnosis. Then appropriate herbal medicine is prescribed.

The theory of the six stages of disease was developed by the physician Chang Chung Ching in his ancient text, *Shang Han*

Lun, the *Treatise on Ailments Attributed to the Cold.* Cold diseases can go through three yang stages and three yin stages.*
Symptoms of the yang stages of a disease manifest themselves early in the illness, while symptoms of the yin stages of disease take longer to develop and progress more slowly. At the beginning (or yang stages) of an illness the patient may have more strength to combat the illness. If a patient becomes weakened by the illness, the disease may progress into the yin stages.

When the yin condition reaches its extreme, death occurs. To prevent this the disease must be checked and the body condition returned to normal at some stage in the development of the disease. The human body can often accomplish this rebalancing by its own devices. At other times medicine must be resorted to.

Since all diseases are the result of an imbalance of yin and yang, it is not necessary to use a different tea for treatment of each disease. However, since there are several stages of disease and differing body qualities, more than a few teas are necessary. For this reason the theory of the stages of disease refers to about sixteen teas.

The Stages of Disease

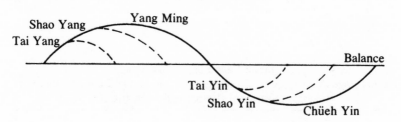

*It should be noted that here yin and yang do not occur in the familiar progression shown in the table on page 34. The pattern here is based on one of several possible configurations of the tripartite divisions of ying yang: big yang (*tai* yang), small yang (*shao* yang), clear yang (yang *ming*), big yin (tai yin), small yin (shao yin), and receding yin (*chüeh* yin). "Clear yang" is a translation of the Chinese term "ming," literally, "bright" or "clear." Here it signifies that stage of disease between small yang and beginning yin. The term "receding yin" is a loose translation of the term "chüeh." Here it is applied to the final yin stage of disease.

Big Yang Stage (Tai Yang)
Disease has not penetrated the body's defenses; it is still in the skin and muscles.

GENERAL SYMPTOMS
fever, strong pulse, headache, stiff shoulders, body pain, cough, chills

SYMPTOMS DENOTING A YIN BODY	TREATMENT
some or all general symptoms and sweating	Kuei chih t'ang

SYMPTOMS DENOTING A BALANCED BODY
some general symptoms, no sweating — Ke ken t'ang

SYMPTOMS DENOTING A YANG BODY
all general symptoms, no sweating — Ma huang t'ang

GENERAL TREATMENT
Half an hour after the administration of herbal tea (t'ang), the patient may eat soft rice porridge. The patient should keep warm, avoid drafts, and eat no animal food, fruit, or sugar.

Note that this first stage is the only instance in which symptoms are differentiated specifically according to body type. As a disease progresses, body type has less and less bearing on the mode of treatment.

Small Yang Stage (Shao Yang)
At this stage the disease is half inside the body and half outside; therefore the symptoms are alternatingly cold and hot.

SYMPTOMS	TREATMENT
strong surface pulse	(Teas for most-yang body quality listed first,
dizziness	descending to less-yang)
bitter taste in mouth	
vomiting	Ta ch'ai hu t'ang
blurred vision	Ch'ai hu chia lung ku mu li t'ang
dry throat	Hsiao ch'ai hu t'ang
	Generally use: Hsiao ch'ai hu t'ang

Clear Yang stage (Yang Ming)

In this stage the disease may enter the meridians of the stomach and intestines.

SYMPTOMS	TREATMENT
hardness of abdomen constipation pulse in wavelike motions	(Teas for most-yang body quality listed first, descending to less-yang)
dry feces	Jun ch'ang t'ang
excessive sweating	Ma tzu jen wan
high fever	Ta ch'eng ch'i t'ang
no fear of cold	Ts'ao ho ch'eng ch'i t'ang
	T'iao wei ch'eng ch'i t'ang
or	Hsiao ch'eng ch'i t'ang
dry feces distended stomach pulse deep and hard mumbling in sleep restlessness constipation thirst	If one of the above teas causes diarrhea, body quality is very yin. Discontinue use of that tea. If diarrhea persists for more than one day, body quality is exceptionally yin. Administer Szu ni t'ang.

Note: Two sets of symptoms are shown here. The same treatment applies for both.

Very often people think that fever, cough, cold, and so on are yin symptoms. This is a serious mistake. Yang diseases are usually very easy to cure, but in extremely yang conditions, such as pneumonia and bronchitis, if a patient is made more yang his condition will rapidly change to yin and he will die quickly.

Big Yin Stage (Tai Yin)

The spleen is affected and the stomach cannot transform liquid food and water.

SYMPTOMS	TREATMENT
quick weak pulse stomach pain distended soft abdomen no thirst vomiting diarrhea	Chen wu t'ang, or Li chung t'ang, or Szu ni t'ang

Small Yin Stage (Shao Yin)

In this stage the disease has entered the heart and kidney. Symptoms may either be empty yang with cold or empty yin with heat.

SYMPTOMS	TREATMENT
empty yang with cold	Chen wu t'ang, or
no vitality	Li chung t'ang, or
cold extremities	Szu ni t'ang
diarrhea, immediately after eating	
vomiting	
empty yin with heat	
restlessness	
diarrhea, not immediately after eating	
sore dry throat	
distended chest	

Note: Treatment for both sets of symptoms is the same.

Receding Yin Stage (Chüeh Yin)

In this stage the disease has damaged all organs. There is heat in the upper torso and cold in the lower torso. The yin has affected the heart governor (pericardium) and the liver. Death may soon follow.

SYMPTOMS	TREATMENT
pain and heat in the throat	Chen wu t'ang
hunger	Li chung t'ang
passing of worms from the abdomen	Szu ni t'ang
vomiting	

As we know, things don't always go according to plan. Occasionally a disease will not progress in the conveniently prescribed manner. When this occurs one must know what course of action to follow. If an earlier yang stage has progressed only partly into a later yang stage, some of the symptoms from the earlier yang stage may remain. In this case the physician treats the earlier yang stage first, then the later stage. For example, if a patient suffers from some symptoms of big yang and some symptoms of small yang, treat big yang first, then small yang. On the other hand, when a patient manifests all the symptoms of two stages simultaneously, the physician treats small yang. In cases in which the patient falls ill with big yang and clear yang simultaneously, the physician treats big yang. Should the patient fall ill with all three yang stages simultaneously, use Hsiao ch'ai hu t'ang when small yang predominates, Pai hu chia jen shen t'ang when clear yang predominates. Generally, use Hsiao ch'ai hu t'ang.

Since treatment for all three yin stages is the same, such considerations need not be taken into account.

A patient whose constitution is yang to begin with will experience the yang stages in rapid succession. Depending on how extreme his yang constitution is, either small yang or clear yang may be experienced quite severely while the other two may pass unnoticed. The yin stages of disease progress more slowly.

Knowledge of the six stages of disease is helpful diagnostically, not only in determining how far a disease has progressed but in judging the progress of the cure. With treatment and improvement the symptoms of earlier stages may reappear as the patient progresses from the yin stages back to the yang stages.

The Five Elements

The five-element theory, wu hsing, represents an attempt to define the interactivity of the body's organs according to an amalgamation of native medical practice and the theory of elements introduced from India. It is a mnemonic for the complex interrelationship of the six organ groups recognized by Chinese medicine, along with the activities of these organs. This theory also serves to correlate information pertaining to symptomology and treatment.

46

Qualities of the Five Elements

	WOOD	FIRE	EARTH	METAL	WATER
Planet	Jupiter	Mars	Saturn	Venus	Mercury
Direction	East	South	Center	West	North
Season	Spring	Summer	(the Change of Seasons)	Autumn	Winter
Color	Blue	Red	Yellow	White	Black
Perverse Climate	Wind	Heat	Moisture	Dryness	Cold
Organ	Liver	Heart	Spleen	Lungs	Kidneys
Sense	Sight	Speech	Taste	Smell	Hearing
Body	Muscles	Pulse	Flesh	Skin	Bones
Part	Nails	Complexion	Lips	Body Hair	Hair
Orifice	Eyes	Ears	Mouth	Nose	Anal-Urinary
Fluid	Tears	Sweat	Lymph	Mucus	Saliva
Sound	Cry	Laugh	Song	Sob	Groan
Psychic Value	Spirit	Conscience	Ideas	(Animal Spirits)	(Will, Ambition)
Emotions	Anger	Joy	Worry	Grief	Fear
Dynamic Energy	Blood	(Psychic Energy)	Strength	Vitality	Will
Governs	Lungs	Kidney	Liver	Heart	Spleen
Grain	Wheat	Millet	Rye	Rice	Beans
Strain	Eyes	Walking	Sitting	Lying Down	Standing

LAWS GOVERNING THE FIVE ELEMENTS

Laws governing the five elements were based on observance of the behavior of various aspects of the "elements" in relation to one another. Like yin yang, from which they are derived, the five elements do not exist independently, but only in relationship to one another. Accordingly, the laws are relative.

Two cycles rule the five elements: The Shen or creative cycle (with its corollary mother-son relationship) and the Kou or destructive cycle. The creative cycle and mother-son relationship lie along the outside of the pentagram. Together they state that each element engenders, nurtures, or gives energy to its neighbor (and all following neighbors), moving in a clockwise direction around the pentagram. This is harmonious change. The

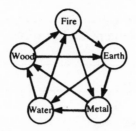

mother-son relationship suggests that as a child is dependent upon its mother for nurture and support, the seasons (elements) emerge and develop one from another. Naturally, movement occurs from summer to fall and so on through the seasons. Thus a change effected in the creative cycle will continue to affect change throughout the cycle in the same direction.

The destructive cycle states that the elements may counteract one another. Moving in a straight line along a leg of the pentagram one encounters configurations which change abruptly from yin to yang. This is not harmonious change. Therefore the term "destructive" applies. Since the destructive cycle is based on unharmonious change, one may cancel a prevailing condition through the use of this cycle. When a cancellation is effected in the destructive cycle, the cycle does not continue but stops after one leg of the pentagram.

The five-element theory is basic to diagnosis. Bodily functions, organs, acupuncture meridians, emotions, even external influences are assigned to the various elements. The five-element theory provides a simple means for remembering the interrelationship of these attributes. In treatment, the five-element theory is employed primarily for acupuncture, but it is also used, though less fundamentally, for herbal medicine.

The mode of herbal treatment is similar to that of acupuncture. For example, an imbalance (i.e., an excess yang or a deficiency yin) in earth may stem from an imbalance in wood via the creative cycle, or a deficiency in metal coupled with an excess in earth may demand the use of a tea to reduce the energy of earth, or to add energy to metal. Which stratagem should be employed will depend upon the diagnostic profile, the symptoms, the pulse diagnosis, and the history of the complaint. A physician may adapt a variety of therapeutic techniques depending upon the situation. Usually five-element teas are used in conjunction with acupuncture to supplement and reinforce treatment.

ELEMENT	ADD ENERGY	REDUCE ENERGY
Fire	Fu tzu t'ang	Chu ch'ueh t'ang
	Chen wu t'ang	Ta ch'ai hu t'ang
		Ts'ao ho ch'eng ch'i t'ang
		Ta ch'eng ch'i t'ang
Earth	Kuei p'i t'ang	Yin ch'en kao t'ang
Metal	Li chung t'ang	Ma huang t'ang
Water	Chen wu t'ang	Wu ling t'ang
	Pa wei wan	
Wood	Kuei chih t'ang	Yi kan san
	Hsiao chien chung t'ang	Yin ch'en kao t'ang

Chapter 3
SYMPTOMATIC
MEDICINE
AND THERAPEUTIC
REPERTORY

The ultimate goal of the classical Chinese physician is to prevent illness through the regulation of energy. According to the laws of Chinese medicine this is called energetic medicine. Ideally this is accomplished through the establishment of a dynamic equilibrium among the forces of a patient's constitutional proclivity and of his immediate condition, and the timely external forces such as climate, geography, and so on. However, this is an ideal and it assumes a healthy patient from the outset of treatment.

More often than not a patient consults a physician only after a complaint has developed. At this point energetic medicine may not meet the patient's desire for immediate relief from his symptoms. There are also cases in which symptoms have developed to the extent that they pose a greater threat to the organism than the original energetic cause of the symptom (i.e., spontaneous eruptions of the skin that have become infected). In addition there are cases in which a symptom arising from a relatively superficial imbalance will affect the body in such a way as to prevent treatment by energetic treatment (i.e., severe constipation arising from external conditions such as climate and diet).

For all these situations Chinese medicine employs treatment to remove the conditions that prevent straightforward treatment according to the laws of energetic medicine. This kind of treatment is called symptomatic medicine. Once those conditions are removed, treatment is returned to the realm of energetic medicine to eradicate the original imbalance (or new imbalances that may have arisen during the crises and treatment). This phase of treatment is then followed by periodic checkups and health maintenance.

Symptomatic medicine is an important branch of Chinese medicine. Its study and practice is extremely useful, and its employment is often indispensable in clinical practice. But it is always subsidiary to energetic medicine. A traditional doctor will never contradict the laws of energetic medicine for the sake of symptomatic treatment. On the contrary, he will most often devise a method of treatment that works symptomatically *through* the laws of energetic medicine.

Abnormal Metabolism

Diabetes
  Pa wei wan
  Ta ch'ai hu t'ang
Hyperhidrosis
  Fang yi huang t'ang
Obesity Disorders
  Fang feng t'ung t'ang
  Ta ch'ai hu t'ang

Anal Conditions

Piles, Protocele, Bleeding of Hemorrhoids
  Yi tzu t'ang
  Tang kuei t'iao yao san
  Pu chung yi ch'i t'ang

Blood Disorders

Anemia
Tang kuei t'iao yao san
Pu chung yi ch'i t'ang
Anemia with Parasites
San wei che ku ts'ai t'ang
Lien chu t'ang
Blood Stagnation
Ts'ao ho ch'eng ch'i t'ang
Epistaxis
San huang hsieh hsin t'ang
Hemmorhage, Blood in the Sputum, Vomiting Blood, Epistaxis,
Bleeding Hemorrhoids, Postpartum Bleeding
Huang lien chieh tu t'ang
San huang hsieh hsin t'ang
Pu chung yi ch'i t'ang
Phlebitis
Kuei chih fu ling wan
Ta huang mu tan t'ang
Pyorrhea
Ts'ao ho ch'eng ch'i t'ang

Dermatological Conditions

Bruises and Contusions
Kuei chih fu ling t'ang
Comedones
Kuei chih fu ling wan
Shih wei t'iao tu t'ang
Eczema
Shih wei t'iao tu t'ang
Kuei chih fu ling wan
Frostbite
Tang kuei szu ni chia wu chu yü shêng chiang t'ang
Tang kuei t'iao yao san

52

Hair Loss
  Ch'ai hu chia lung ku mu li t'ang
Keratosis of the Palm
  Tang kuei szu ni chia wu chu yü shêng chiang t'ang
Skin Itching
  Huang lien chieh tu t'ang
  Chi tzu pai pi t'ang
Warts
  Ma hsing yi kan t'ang
  Shih wei t'iao tu t'ang

Digestive Conditions

Acute Gastritis
  Huang ken chieh tu t'ang
Appendicitis
  Ta huang mu tan t'ang
  Kuei chih ch'ia shao yao t'ang
Dysentery
  Ke ken t'ang
  Ta ch'ai hu t'ang
  Ta huang mu t'ang
  Chen wu t'ang
Enteritis, Loose Bowels with Gripping Pain, Diarrhea
  Kuei chih chia shao yao t'ang
  Chen wu t'ang
  Fu tzu t'ang
  Szu ni t'ang
  Li chung t'ang
Food Poisoning
  Yin ch'en kao t'ang
Gastroptosis, Gastric Atony, Gastric Dilation
  Shao yao kan ts'ao t'ang
  Pan hsia hsieh hsin t'ang
  Ta ch'ai hu t'ang
Hepatitis
  Yin chen wu ling t'ang

Jaundice, Cholecystitis, Cholelithiasis
   Yin chen wu ling t'ang
   Ta ch'ai hu t'ang
   Chih tzu kan lien t'ang
Liver Trouble
   Ta ch'ai hu t'ang
   Hsiao ch'ai hu t'ang
Nausea, Vomiting
   Pan hsia hou p'o t'ang
   Pan hsia hsieh hsin t'ang
Nervous Esophagostenosis (Stricture of the Throat)
   Pan hsia hou p'o t'ang
Peritonitis
   Chen wu t'ang
   Huang chü chien chung t'ang
Poor Appetite
   Pan hsia hsieh hsin t'ang
   P'ing wei san
   Hsiao ch'ai wu t'ang
Stomach-ache, Stomach Cramp, Heartburn, Gastritis
   Huang lien chieh tu t'ang
   Li mu t'ang
   Fu ling t'ang
Stomach Neurosis
   Pan hsia hsieh hsin t'ang
Stomatitis
   Ping wei san
   Huang lien chieh tu t'ang
Vitamin Deficiency
   Chi ming san chia tu ling t'ang

Gynecological Disorders

Agalactia
   Ke ken t'ang
   P'u kung ying t'ang

Cold Constitution
  Tang kuei t'iao yao san
  Kuei chi fu ling wan
  Tang kuei szu ni chia wu chu yü shêng chiang t'ang
  Pa wei wan
Disorders of the Female Reproductive Organs, Leucorrhea, Conditions Related to Childbirth
  Kuei chih fu ling t'ang
  Tang kuei t'iao yao san
  Ts'ao ho ch'eng ch'i t'ang
  Lung tan hsieh kan t'ang
Impure Blood
  Kuei chih fu ling wan
Mastitis
  Ke ken t'ang
Menopause, Female Dizziness
  Ch'ai hu kuei chih t'ang
  Ts'ao ho ch'eng ch'i t'ang
  Tang kuei t'iao yao san
Morning Sickness
  Pan hsia hou p'o t'ang
  Pan hsia hsieh hsin t'ang
Pregnancy with History of Miscarriage
  Kuei chih fu ling wan
Uterine Cysts, Tumors
  Ts'ao ho ch'eng ch'i t'ang
Vaginitis, Pudendal Eczema, Pruritus
  Lung tan hsieh kan t'ang

Heart Conditions

Heart Disease, Endocarditis, Valvular Disease
  Ch'ai hu kuei kan chiang t'ang
  Tang kuei t'iao yao san
  Lung kuei shu kan t'ang

High Blood Pressure, Arteriosclerosis, Hemiplegia
Ch'ai hu chia lung ku mu li t'ang
Fang feng t'ung sheng san
San huang hsieh hsin t'ang
Ta ch'ai hu t'ang

Low Blood Pressure, Abnormal Blood Pressure
Tang kuei t'iao yao san
Pu chung yi ch'i t'ang

Tachycardia
Ch'ai hu ch'ia lung ku mu li t'ang
Chiu wei pin lang t'ang
Lung kuei shu kan t'ang

Nerve and Motor Disorders

Dizziness, Vertigo, Heavy-headedness
Hsiang su t'ang
Tang kuei t'iao yao san

Epilepsy
Ch'ai hu chia lung ku mu li t'ang
Kan huang hsieh hsin t'ang
Ke ken t'ang
Kuei chih fu ling t'ang

Headache, Hot Fit, Tinnitus Aurium
Hsiang su t'ang
  a. Headache due to blood stagnation
    Ts'ao ho ch'eng ch'i t'ang
  b. Headache with pain on inside of the head
    Tang kuei t'iao yao san
  c. Headache accompanied by thirst and decreased
    urination
    Wu ling t'ang
  d. Headache accompanied by blood congestion
    San huang hsieh hsin t'ang
  e. Headache accompanied by fever
    Ma huang t'ang
    Ke ken t'ang

    f. Headache accompanied by dull pain
         Hsiao ch'ai hu t'ang
         Kuei chih t'ang

Parkinson's Disease
    Hsiao ch'eng ch'i t'ang

Ophthalmological Conditions

Conjunctivitis, Lacryoadenitis
    Ke ken t'ang
    Hsiao ch'ing lung t'ang
Cataracts
    Chu hua t'ang
    Pa wei wan
Myopia, Hyperopia, Astigmatism
    Ling kuei shu kan t'ang

Otorhinolaryngological Conditions

Sore Throat
    Chieh keng t'ang
    Pan hsia hsieh hsin t'ang
Tonsillitis
    Ke ken t'ang
Toothache
    Li hsiao san

Pediatric Disorders

Autointoxication
    Li chung t'ang
Cervical Lymphadenitis
    Ch'ai hu kuei chih t'ang

Eneuresis, Diuresis
   Hsiao chien chung t'ang
   Pa wei wan
Infantile Asthma
   Ma hsing yi kan t'ang
Infantile Neurosis, Night Crying, Night Fright
   Hsiao chien chung t'ang
Scrofulosis, underdevelopment
   Hsaio ch'ai hu t'ang
   Pa ching yi ch'i t'ang
   Hsiao chien chung t'ang

Respiratory Conditions

Asthma (Bronchial)
   Hsiao ch'ing lung t'ang
   Ma hsing yi kan t'ang
Cardiac Asthma
   Pan hsia hou p'o t'ang
   Mu fang i t'ang
Cold
   Ke ken t'ang
   Ch'ai hu kuei chih t'ang
   Ma huang t'ang
   Hsiao ch'ai hu t'ang
   Su tzu chiang ch'i t'ang
   Pa wei wan
   Hsiang su t'ang
   Kuei chih t'ang
Cough, Bronchitis
   Hsiao ch'ing lung t'ang
   Hsiao ch'ai hu t'ang
   Mai men tung t'ang
   Ling kan chiang wei hsin hsia jen t'ang
   Ma huang t'ang

Dry Cough
  Ch'ai hu kuei kan chiang t'ang
Hemoptysis
  Mai men tung t'ang
  Huang lien chieh tu t'ang
  Chih kan ts'ao t'ang
Pleurisy
  Ch'ai hu kuei chih t'ang
  Hsiao ch'ai hu t'ang
Sinusitis
  Ke ken t'ang
Whooping Cough
  Hsiao ch'ing lung t'ang
  Kan mai ta tsao t'ang
  Ta ch'ing lung t'ang
Pneumonia
  Ta ch'ing lung t'ang
  Ta ch'ai hu t'ang
  Hsao ch'ai hu t'ang

Urinary, Genital Troubles

Abnormal Urination, Frequent and Infrequent Urination
  Chu ling t'ang
  Wu ling t'ang
  Pa wei wan
  Ling kuei shu kan t'ang
  Kan mai ta tsao t'ang
Atrophied Kidney
  Pa wei wan
Edema, Swelling
  Wu ling t'ang
  Pan hsia hou p'o t'ang
Kidney Disease
  Wu ling t'ang
  Pa wei wan
  Ta ch'eng ch'i t'ang
  Fang feng t'ung shêng san

Loss of Vitality, Impotence, Sexual Neurasthenia
   Pa wei wan
   Ch'ai hu ch'ai lung ku mu li t'ang
   Ta ch'ai hu t'ang
Nephritis, Nephrosis
   Wu ling t'ang
   Chu ling t'ang
   Tang kuei szu ni chia wu chu yü shêng chiang t'ang
   Pa wei wan
Nocturnal Micturition, Nocturnal Diuresis
   Hsiao chien chung t'ang
   Pa wei wan
Venereal Disease
   Shih wei t'iao tu t'ang
   Lung tan hsieh kan t'ang
      a. syphilis
         Hsing ch'uan chieh tu t'ang
      b. gonorrhea
         Chu ling t'ang (+ Yin chen 4. ch'ien)
         Wu ling t'ang (+ Yin chen 4. ch'ien)

Miscellaneous

Adynamia, Debility, Weight Loss, Anemia, Night Sweating
   Hsiao ch'ai hu t'ang
   Wu chi san
Constitutional Improvement
   Hsiao ch'ai hu t'ang
   Ta ch'ai hu t'ang
Fatigue and Weariness
   Chiu wei pin lang t'ang
   Ta ch'ai hu t'ang
   Pa wei wan
   Chen wu t'ang
   Kan mai ta tsao t'ang
   Pu chung yi ch'i t'ang

Hernia
    Hsiao chien chung t'ang
    Ch'ai hu kuei chih t'ang
Mental Disorders
    Pan hsia hsieh hsin t'ang
    Suan tsao jen t'ang
    Tang kuei szu ni chia wu chu yü shêng chiang t'ang
    Ch'ai hu chia lung ku mu li t'ang
Worms and Parasites
    San wei che ku ts'ai t'ang
    Ke ken t'ang

Chapter 4
DIAGNOSIS AND DISCHARGE

Oriental diagnosis always considers sickness a condition of the whole body, even though isolated symptoms may appear in one area or another. Oriental medicine does not hold with the germ theory of disease. (However, it is recognized that germs are often the vehicles of certain diseases.) Nor does Oriental medicine hold that an external condition alone can bring about disease in a healthy body. Instead it holds that body condition is the primary factor contributing to either health or disease. Therefore isolation of external causes is not necessary for treatment and prevention of disease. Instead, the internal condition of the body must be regulated according to the yin yang theory of the way of nature. Oriental diagnosis puts primary emphasis on judging the yin yang condition of the body.

Oriental diagnosis employs four methods: looking, listening and smelling, questioning, and touching. Of the four, *looking* is by far the most important, as it is almost universally applicable. It may be used for babies, unconscious people, uncooperative patients, and in general anyone who cannot or will not speak—these all being cases in which questioning diagnosis is not possible. Similarly, it can be used for patients who have an arm injured or missing, thus rendering pulse taking—one type of touching diagnosis—impossible. Looking diagnosis may be used at any time, under any circumstances, with or without a patient's cooperation or even his knowledge that he is being diagnosed. It is said that those who have mastered the art of looking are gods.

Indeed, it may seem to be so. One who has mastered this art can look at a person's face and see his past and probable future reflected there as clearly as if it were written in a book. Thus the study of physiognomy, skin colors, texture, and other facial signs are important diagnostic criteria, and are found to be correlated in detail with pulse palpation and other forms of diagnosis in Chinese pathology and treatment. The most important element in this type of diagnosis, however, is the general impression gained at first glance. This must be held in mind throughout the entire diagnosis. Second, analytical yin yang diagnosis must be made and unified as a whole. The two must then be considered together before a final diagnosis is reached. If both extremes of yin and yang exist simultaneously, much caution must be exercised in reaching a diagnosis and prescribing treatment.

To make a first-glance diagnosis, one must consider the body characteristics which appear most prominent; energy, shape, and color. These must be classified according to yin yang, empty full, and the five-elements theories. Any pertinent information must be abstracted from these theories. Though it is presented here in a broken down and conceptualized order, one should remember that in practice this phase of diagnosis must be performed intuitively rather than analytically. A physician should not look at a patient and then say to himself, "Hmm, his face color is rather yellow. If I remember correctly, that's pancreas and spleen." The entire phase must be executed at a single glance without hesitation or afterthought. It goes without saying that extensive analytical training is necessary if one is to become proficient at this type of diagnosis.

The basic body characteristics are listed below with their yin yang, empty full, and five-element classifications.

Yin Yang

	YIN	YANG
energy	passive	active
shape	narrow, tall	broad, short

Empty Full

	YIN EMPTY	YIN FULL	YANG EMPTY	YANG FULL
energy	passive	passive	active	active
color	pale	yellow	tan	red
shape	thin	plump	wiry	heavy

The Five Elements

	WOOD	FIRE	EARTH	METAL	WATER
indication	liver disease	heart disease	spleen-pancreas disease	lung disease	kidney disease
color	blue	red	yellow	pale	dark

The analytical approach is to scrutinize every part of the body, noting its individual yin yang quality as delineated by appearance while simultaneously making reference to the various internal organs and viscera associated with these body parts. For instance, the nose is thought to reflect the condition of the heart. Red is a yang color. Therefore a prominent red nose usually indicates a heart that is too yang.

The next most important method is *listening and smelling*. Like looking, listening and smelling may be employed without a patient's cooperation or knowledge. However, it is somewhat more limited than looking in that one must get rather close to a patient to apply this method. It is said that a master of the art can often diagnose a patient by entering his house and smelling the air or by hearing him speak only a few words. It is also said that one who has mastered this system is a sage.

The Five Sounds

Shouting	Liver, Gall Bladder
Speaking	Heart, Small Intestines
Singing	Spleen, Stomach
Crying	Lungs, Colon
Groaning	Kidneys, Bladder

SHOUTING   Those who shout frequently are usually quick to become angry. They invariably suffer from liver and gall bladder troubles.

SPEAKING   Persons who talk incessantly without pause or purpose and those who stutter usually suffer from heart trouble. Those who speak clearly and express themselves eloquently with few words have a healthy and well-toned heart.

SINGING   Those who sing well have a good stomach and spleen. Those who sing incessantly or seem to have a singsong quality to their voices often suffer from spleen or stomach disorders.

CRYING   Those who cry often and those who pine and sigh suffer from lung troubles.

GROANING   Groaning, moaning, yawning, and snoring all reflect bad kidneys.

When only symptoms for degenerative conditions are given in the list above (i.e., kidneys), the absence of such sounds indicates the absence of a degenerative condition. It should be kept in mind, however, that while this method of diagnosis may not reveal a symptom of degeneration another one may.

The Five Odors

Rancid	Liver, Gall Bladder
Scorched	Heart, Small Intestines
Fragrant	Spleen, Stomach
Rotten	Lungs, Colon
Putrid	Kidney, Bladder

The presence of any of the odors except the fragrant odor indicates a degenerative condition of the corresponding organs. The fragrant odor indicates a very well-conditioned stomach and spleen.

Questioning diagnosis involves asking the patient for his own complaints, explanations, and opinions. According to Oriental medical ethics, if a patient complains that he is sick, he must be diagnosed as ill even if no symptoms are found. The physician must then reconsider the case himself or seek the help of a more skilled diagnostician. In respect to this point, perhaps modern medicine and traditional Oriental medicine are not dissimilar. But with regard to the opposite condition, the two are greatly at odds. Oriental medicine holds that if a patient feels he is well, even though degenerative symptoms are present and made known to him, then he must not be considered sick. Though this may seem strange to modern ears, understanding this point is paramount to understanding Oriental medicine. Questioning is a most important phase of diagnosis because it establishes the patient's mental attitude toward his condition. This information is quite helpful to the physician because it is a good indication of how much cooperation can be expected from the patient. Considerable tact must be exercised in applying this method, both in asking questions and in interpreting answers. Patients' explanations are not accepted verbatim but always weighed with information provided by the other systems of diagnosis.

Questions should be asked to reveal information concerning aches, pains, temperature, chills, urination, defecation, menstruation, appetite, and sleep. Any abnormality is a clue to the nature and origin of the illness. Yang symptoms are:

> aches and pains
> stiffness
> temperature and chills
> sweating
> inability to sleep

Yin symptoms are:

> loss of appetite
> excessive sleeping and easy tiring

Information concerning urination and defecation is most important in questioning diagnosis. This provides a very pragmatic and recent diagnosis of the patient's condition.

A healthy male eating a well-balanced diet should urinate four or five times a day. A healthy female eating a balanced diet should urinate three or four times a day except during pregnancy, when urination occurs more frequently due to compression of the bladder. More frequent urination indicates a yin condition. Healthy urine should be the color of beer. If it is darker, the person's most recent condition is too yang; if lighter, too yin.

A child's urine should, of course, be thinner than an adult's and a child may urinate much more frequently.

The feces should be firm, buoyant, large, and not extremely putrid smelling. If the feces smells putrid, there is stomach or intestinal trouble. If the feces are loose and green in color the condition is yin. If the feces are hard and dark, the condition is usually too yang. The patient may be suffering from constipation. Though constipation is usually a yang condition, there is a yin type of constipation. In that case the feces are hard and firm but they are not glossy as they usually are; instead they are rather dull.

Urination shows the most recent condition, that which has been established in the past few hours. Defecation shows the condition that has been established within the past few days.

Touching diagnosis is the least idealistic and most direct and pragmatic of the four methods. This method gives the most immediate diagnosis of a patient's condition. Since it is the most accurate it is used to verify the findings of the other methods. It is most important for beginners and those whose command of the other forms has not matured. It is said that one who has mastered this system is a skillful physician.

Touching diagnosis employs four methods:

> feeling for temperature and water content
> palpating the abdomen
> palpating diagnostic acupuncture points
> reading the pulses

The above methods are listed from the most general one reading down to the most specialized practice. They are used in the same order.

TEMPERATURE AND WATER

With this method the physician feels the forehead, hand, and/or foot. High temperature and dryness of the hands and feet are yang symptoms. A low or slightly high temperature and wet hands or feet indicate a yin condition.

ABDOMINAL PALPATION

The abdomen should have a good complexion and be resilient, neither too hard nor too soft. The patient should experience no unusual pains or sensations there.

Stiffness or pulsation in the abdomen may be either yin or yang; other symptoms must be considered. In most cases stiffness in the upper abdomen is a symptom of a yang condition. If the lower part of the abdomen is very soft, this is a symptom of a yin condition.

The skin on the abdomen should not be loose and fatty, so that it could easily be pinched, nor should it be too thick or hard. Both loose, fatty skin and thick, hard skin are yang symptoms, usually attributable to consumption of animal foods. A thin skin is a sign of yin condition.

Fullness of the abdomen may show yin and/or yang causes. If the patient has a strong pulse and is constipated, the fullness is a yang symptom. If the pulse is weak and there is no constipation, the fullness is a yin symptom. When the fullness occurs in the lower part of the abdomen and is accompanied by excessive urination, rushes of blood to the head, and pain upon palpation, the cause is blood stagnation. This may be attributed to an excess of both yin and yang factors.

The sound of water upon palpation is a sign of gastritis. The sound of thunder or howling wind is a sign of a yin condition.

DIAGNOSTIC ACUPUNCTURE POINTS

The palpation of diagnostic points is employed to reveal the hypoactivity or hyperactivity of the organs corresponding to the various points. Once a point has been located, it is pressed lightly with the tip of the index finger or the fleshy ball of the thumb. If pain is felt, it is an indication that the organ in question is hypoactive—yin. If no pain is felt, heavier pressure is applied. If pain is then felt, it is an indication that the organ in question is hyperactive—yang. No pain in either case indicates that the corresponding organ is in good tone. This method of diagnosis is developed extensively in conjunction with the study of acupuncture.

PULSES

The pulses show an immediate reflection of the condition of the internal organs. When checking the pulses it is most important to feel for the strength of the pulse. The frequency of the pulse is a secondary factor and it need only be judged relatively fast or slow. It is not necessary to establish the precise number of beats within a given period of time. Strength is a yang factor. Slowness is a yin factor. Combining these qualities, four possible types of pulses may be derived: quick and strong—too yang; slow and strong—yang; quick and weak—yin; slow and weak—too yin.

Pulsation is measured at the wrist by pressing down over the radial artery with the index, middle, and ring fingers. Two pulses are read with each finger, a superficial pulse and a deep pulse. Six different pulses are located on each arm, making a total of twelve pulses in all.

While one is reading the pulse the fingers should be held at a 90-degree angle to the radial artery while the patient's palm is bent backward slightly. This procedure is essential for a clear reading. The positioning of the fingers is relative to the height of the physician and his patient. If the patient is the same height as or smaller than the physician, the fingers are held so that they touch. If the patient is taller, the fingers are spaced slightly farther apart. The first step in reading the pulses is to establish the mean pulse quality. Feeling with all three fingers at once, press to a median depth and judge the pulse. This is the median pulse. The individual pulses are measured relative to this one. The superficial pulse is read by pressing lightly, just enough so that one may feel the pulse. The deep pulse is read by pressing deeply until the blood flow is almost stopped. Upon first experimentation differences in the pulses may be difficult to discern. Only after practice do these become clear. Beginners are traditionally instructed to try at least one hundred pulses before assuming some small understanding of the practice. Like point palpation, this method is usually more extensively developed with the study of acupuncture.

Discharge

After a period of treatment a patient may show certain symptoms which would be considered signs of illness under any other circumstances. Provided that these symptoms are of a specified nature and follow an orderly pattern of development, they are perfectly natural. The process of their appearance and disappearance is called discharge. It indicates that a cure is taking effect. The symptoms are caused by the body's activity in ridding itself of excesses. Discharge occurs in three consecutive stages. Though any one stage may manifest itself more strongly than the others, each stage should occur in its time, at least to some degree. *Deviation from this orderly pattern, or the occurrence of severe symptoms which do not subside quickly, must be construed as a worsening condition of disease.*

STAGES OF DISCHARGE

FIRST STAGE. The tongue may change color and small white "pimples" may occur toward the back of the tongue. A violet color indicates a yin discharge. White or yellow indicates yang. The hands and/or feet may ache.

SECOND STAGE. The first-stage symptoms subside. The tongue discharge moves forward on the tongue. The patient may complain of a heated feeling though no temperature is present. There may be pain in the throat and/or genital regions.

Yang people feel this stage strongly. Since they discharge more easily and more quickly, yang people finish most of their discharging in this stage. Yin people do not discharge so easily and consequently they are usually not affected much by this stage.

THIRD AND FINAL STAGE. The symptoms of the second stage subside. The tongue discharge moves to the tip of the tongue or may subside altogether. Pain may be felt in the abdomen, extremities, or head (headaches). In this final stage there is great danger due to severe headaches that sometimes occur. Often these are accompanied by cloudy thinking and a feeling of despair. The patient may lose sight of what is taking place and do something contrary to treatment. Careful observation is recommended in cases in which this stage is intense. This stage is felt most strongly by very yin people.

During or after this stage, the patient may pass shiny, dark or black, elastic fecal material similar to that passed by a newborn baby just after it begins to nurse. This is fecal matter that has been in the intestines for a long time because of general dysfunction of the intestines and disharmony of the body.

In some cases no outward signs of discharge occur, except that the diseased condition subsides. When the patient is relatively healthy or the disease slight, this is normal.

Chapter 5
TEAS AND OTHER HERBAL PREPARATIONS:
Teas Most Commonly Used in the Chinese Pharmacopeia

(In Romanized Alphabetical Order with Annotated Chinese Characters)

Approximately 120 prescriptions make up the basic repertory of Chinese herbal medicine. These are applied through one of three methods of preparation.

Wan (pill). The herbs are ground into a fine powder and mixed with a binding agent such as honey, then rolled into pellets. These are then taken with boiled water or warm water.

San (powder). The herbs are ground into a fine powder which is dissolved in boiled water or warm water.

T'ang (soup). The herbs are put into a nonmetallic (i.e., glass, ceramic, enamel, or earthenware) vessel with three cups of cold water. This is brought to a rolling boil, then allowed to simmer until only one and a half cups remain, about 25–30 minutes. After the liquid is strained off and drunk, the herbs can be used again in the same manner the following day, provided that there are no soluble ingredients. After the herbs are brewed twice they must be discarded.

Prescriptions are usually taken once a day, preferably in the morning on an empty stomach, and should not be followed by any food for one-half hour.

71

Because weights, recipes, and even choice of teas will always differ slightly from one physician to another, there can never be a letter perfect exposition of this repertory. However, there can be a somewhat representational exposition with which most herbalists would agree most of the time. This is what the author has striven for here.

The weights given here are not the same as the original measures given by Muramoto in his handwritten notes. After conferral with a number of Chinese herbalists it was decided that these measures were overly conservative and so in all cases these measurements have been increased by a factor of approximately three. For example, where Muramoto had given:

Ch'ai hu ch'ia lung ku mu li t'ang
5 gr. ch'ai hu
4 gr. pan hsia
3 gr. fu ling
--etc--

the author has altered this to read:

Ch'ai hu ch'ia lung ku mu li t'ang
5 ch'ien ch'ai hu
4 ch'ien pan hsia
3 ch'ien fu ling
--etc--

In addition to these changes, the measures have been converted from the metric system to the Chinese measuring system. This should facilitate the use of this text by Chinese pharmacists who, for the most part, are more familiar with these terms. If the reader should wish to convert these back to the metric system the following table may be used:

1 chin = 16 liang [Chinese ounce] = 500 gm.
1 liang = 10 ch'ien = 31.2 gm.
1 ch'ien = 10 fen = 3.12 gm.
2 chin = 1 kg. = 1000 gm.

Many of the entries in this section include conditions limiting the use of a particular tea. These are listed at the bottom of each entry in the following form:

Conditions: for yin people; may be used one month.

The absence of such a note may be taken as an indication that there are no limiting factors regarding use of that particular tea.

Finally, a word of advice on the subject of doses and usage from *A Barefoot Doctor's Manual*:

"When drugs are given, one must take a scientific attitude and a creative approach at the same time. Information on the patient with respect to sex, age, general health, severity and duration of illness, climatic factors, etc., must be considered and analyzed.

"Generally speaking, the amount of medication prescribed for a healthy individual may be greater than that for a weaker person; greater for a young adult than an aged person or child; also greater for a man than a woman. Smaller dosages are given for a milder disease, and larger doses for more severe illnesses. Chronic diseases should be treated slowly [prolonged] with smaller doses, and acute ailments should be given heavy dose(s) in an abrupt attempt to save the patient and dispel evil [effects of illness]. Dosage of drugs with strong or toxic properties should be strictly controlled—from smaller to larger doses. Excessive use of bitter and cooling drugs are harmful to the stomach and spleen. Peppery and hot drugs should be given with care to patients with deficient and heat-dominating constitution. Purgative drugs that disrupt energy and blood should be avoided by pregnant women or used only with care. Few heat-type drugs should be used in the summer, and few cold-type drugs in the winter. Drugs containing light porous materials such as flowers and leaves should be used in small amounts, and those containing minerals and shells, in larger amounts. Aromatics to restore 'breath' should be used sparingly, and juicy drugs to restore 'taste' should be used more heavily. What has been described are only general principles prescribing drug use. In actual practice consider actual conditions and prescribe flexibly when needed."

Ch'ai hu chia lung ku mu li t'ang
Saikokaryukotsuboreito

3 ch'ien	ch'ai hu
4	pan hsia
3	fu ling
3	kuei
2.5	huang ch'in
2.5	tsao
2.5	shêng chiang
2.5	jen shen
2.5	lung ku
2.5	mu li
1	ta huang

柴胡加龍骨牡蠣湯
柴胡 三爻
半夏 四爻
茯苓 三爻
桂枝 三爻半
黄芩 三爻半
大棗 三爻半
生薑 三爻半
人參 三爻半
龍骨 三爻半
牡蠣 三爻半
大黄 一爻

PROPERTIES: warming; discharges excess energy (chi); hypotensive; mild laxative; treats various yang disorders of the circulatory system such as cerebral hemorrhage, heat valve disorders, and hardening of the arteries; treats various mental disorders attributed to hypertension such as hysteria, insomnia, inability to concentrate; benefits the nervous and glandular systems; promotes sexual vitality; treats impotence; treats epilepsy; treats yang stomach disorders; treats progressive baldness.

CONDITIONS: for yang people.

Ch'ai hu kuei chih t'ang
Saikokeishito

5 ch'ien	ch'ai hu
4	pan hsia
2.5	kuei
2	huang ch'in
2	jen shen
2	shao yao
2	shêng chiang
2	tsao
1.5	kan ts'ao

柴胡桂枝湯
柴胡 五爻
半夏 四爻
桂枝 二爻半
黄芩 三爻
人參 三爻
芍藥 三爻
生薑 三爻
大棗 三爻
甘草 二爻半

PROPERTIES: warming; treats common cold and influenza; treats stomach disorders and duodenal ulcers; treats asthma; treats bed-wetting; treats gallstones; occasionally employed for epilepsy or nervous system disorders.

Ch'ai hu kuei kan chiang t'ang
Saikokishikankyoto

6 ch'ien	ch'ai hu
3	kuei
3	kua lou ken
3	huang ch'in
3	mu li
2	kan chiang
2	kan ts'ao

柴胡桂干羌湯

甘 干 牡 黄 瓜 桂 柴胡
草 羌 蠣 芩 呂根 皮 胡
爻 爻 爻 爻 爻 爻 爻

PROPERTIES: treats most disorders rooted in the chest, including heart palpitations, difficult breathing, tightness, bronchitis, and pneumonia; relieves alternating hot and cold flashes; treats insomnia; treats malaria.

CONDITIONS: for rather yin people; may be used for one month.

Che ch'ung yin
Sesshoin

3 ch'ien	mu tan pi
3	hsiung ch'iung
3	shao yao
3	kuei
5	t'ao jen
5	tang kuei
2	yen hu so
2	niu hsi
1	huang hua

折衝飲

紅 牛 延 當 桃 桂 芍 川 牡
花 膝 胡索 歸 仁 枝 藥 芎 丹皮
爻 爻 爻 爻 爻 爻 爻 爻 爻

PROPERTIES: hemocathartic; vasotonic; analgesic; treats gynecopathy, especially disorders arising from childbirth; treats menstrual disorders and pains; stops hemorrhaging after childbirth; relieves itching in the vagina.

CONDITIONS: for yang people.

Che ch'ung yin (alternative)
  Sesshoin

3 ch'ien	mu tan pi
3	hsiung ch'iung
3	shao yao
3	kuei
5	t'ao jen
5	tang kuei
2	su mu
2	niu hsi
1	huang hua

PROPERTIES: hemocathartic; vasotonic; treats gynecopathy, especially disorders arising after childbirth; treats menstrual disorders; stops hemorrhaging at childbirth; relieves itching vagina.

CONDITIONS: for yang people; this tea is a stronger hemocathartic than its alternative.

Chen wu t'ang
  Shinbuto

5 ch'ien	fu ling
3	shao yao
3	shêng chiang
3	ts'ang chu
0.5	fu tzu

PROPERTIES: diuretic; sudorific.

Chi ming san ch'ia fu ling san
  Keimeisan

4 ch'ien	pin lang tzu
3	ming cha
3	shêng chiang
2.5	chü p'i
2.5	chieh keng
1	su yeh
1	wu chu yü
6	fu ling

PROPERTIES: promotes growth of beneficial intestinal flora; treats vitamin B complex deficiency.

CONDITIONS: for very yang people this tea is more effective than Chiu wei pin lang t'ang.

Chia wei hsiao yao san
Kamishoyosan

3 ch'ien	tang kuei
3	shao yao
3	ts'ang chu
3	fu ling
3	ch'ai hu
2	kan ts'ao
2	mu tan pi
2	chih tzu mien
1	shêng chiang
1	p'u ho

加味逍遙散

紫 茯 尤 芍 當
胡 苓   藥 歸
三 三 三 三 三
爻 爻 爻 爻 爻

薄 生 山 牡 甘
荷 毛 梔 丹 草
  子 皮
一 一 一 二 三
爻 爻 爻 爻 爻

PROPERTIES: treats liver disorders; treats mental disorders, including short temper, insomnia, and migraine headaches; treats menstrual disorders; treats bladder disorders; treats eczema; treats hepatitis.

CONDITIONS: for yin people.

Chieh keng t'ang
Kikyoto

2 ch'ien	chieh keng
3	kan ts'ao

桔梗湯

甘 桔
草 梗
一 二
爻 爻

PROPERTIES: expectorant; treats laryngitis, tonsillitis, and sore throat.

CONDITIONS: for yang people; use for short time only.

Chih kan ts'ao t'ang
  Shakanzoto

3 ch'ien	chih kan ts'ao
3	shêng chiang
3	kuei
3	ma jen
3	tsao
3	jen shen
6	ti huang
6	mai men tung
2	a chiao

炙甘草湯

PROPERTIES: cardiac stimulant; produces a strong, steady heartbeat; treats yin heart pace disorders such as weak, racing, or irregular heartbeat.

CONDITIONS: although any type of person may use this tea, it is especially good for yin people.

Chih tzû kan lien t'ang
  Shishikanrento

3 ch'ien	chih tzû mien
1	huang lien
4	kan ts'ao

梔子甘連湯

PROPERTIES: stomachic; treats stomach and duodenal disorders, including ulcers.

Chih tzû pai pi t'ang
  Shishihakuhito

3 ch'ien	chih tzû mien
2	huang po
1	kan ts'ao

梔子柏皮湯

PROPERTIES: cooling; treats stomach disorders; treats jaundice accompanied by fever; treats itchy skin diseases.

Ch'ing chieh lien ch'ih t'ang
  Keikairengyoto

2 ch'ien	tang kuei
2	shao yao
2	ch'ing chieh
2	lien ch'iao
2	fang feng
2	hsiung ch'iung
2	ch'ai hu
2	chih shih
2	huang ch'in
2	chih tzû mien
2	pai chih
2	chieh keng
1	kan ts'ao

荊芥連翹湯

當歸 芍藥 荊芥 連翹 防風 川芎 紫胡

枳實 黄芩 山梔子 白芷 桔梗 甘草

PROPERTIES: stimulates and strengthens the liver; hemostatic; treats epistaxis, sinus and inner ear disorders; hemocathartic; treats acne; treats baldness; treats tuberculosis; treats mental disorders.

Ch'ing je chieh yu t'ang
  Seinetsugentsuto

3 ch'ien	chih tzû mien
3	ts'ang chu
2	hsiung ch'iung
2	hsiang fu tzu
2	ch'ên p'i
1	huang lien
1	kan ts'ao
1	chih shih
0.5	kan chiang
0.5	shêng chiang

清熱解鬱湯

山梔子 蒼朮 川芎 香附子 陳皮

黄連 甘草 枳殼 乾姜 生姜

PROPERTIES: sedative for mental stress; analgesic for upper abdominal pain.

CONDITIONS: not suitable for either very yin or very yang people.

Chiu wei pin lang t'ang
Kuminbinroto

4 ch'ien	pin lang tzu	九味檳榔湯
3	kuei	檳榔子 四
3	chü p'i	桂枝 三
3	hou p'o	橘皮 三
1.5	su yeh	厚朴 三
*1	kan ts'ao	蘇葉 一半
1	ta huang	甘草 一
1	mu hsiang	大黄 一
*1	shêng chiang	木香 一
*3	fu ling	生姜 一
(or) *3	wu chu yü	茯苓 三

PROPERTIES: promotes the growth of beneficial intestinal flora; treats pernicious anemia; treats vitamin B complex deficiency; relieves shallow breathing; treats enlarged heart; relieves swollen legs; treats general weakness; treats weakness of the nervous system. Abundant intestinal flora promotes digestion and absorption of B vitamins; among these B_{12} is particularly important as it enables the body to utilize iron. This tea is used experimentally to treat strange and unrelated symptoms that do not lead to a clear diagnosis.

Chu ling t'ang
Choreito

3 ch'ien	chu ling	猪苓湯
3	fu ling	猪苓 三
3	hua shih	茯苓 三
3	tse hsieh	滑石 三
3	a chiao	澤瀉 三
		阿膠 三

PROPERTIES: induces harmony in the urinary tract; analgesic for urinary discomfort.

CONDITIONS: may be used for one week to three months.

---

*Shêng chiang and kan ts'ao may be used interchangeably or both may be used together, depending on the desired effect. Wu chu yü may be used to replace fu ling if this is desirable. These herbs modify this tea in the following manner; shêng chiang is a stomachic and cardiac stimulant; kan ts'ao is a corrigent and promotes the retention of fluids; fu ling is a diuretic; wu chu yü has a warming effect on the body.

*Fang feng t'ung shêng san
 Bofutsushosan

散 壓 通 風 防

PROPERTIES: diuretic; laxative; diaphoretic; treats yang kidneys and related skin conditions; promotes weight loss.

CONDITIONS: for yang people; may be taken for one to two months. This tea is prepared by mixing approximately one teaspoon of the prepared powder in a glass of water. The solution is then drunk one half-hour before eating or in place of a meal. It may be taken as often as three times daily.

Fang yi huang ch'i t'ang
Boioghito

1 ch'ien	mu fang
5	huang ch'i
3	ts'ang chu
3	shêng chiang
3	tsao
1.5	kan ts'ao

PROPERTIES: diuretic; emmenagogue; treats joint disorders and discomfort; antisudorific; promotes weight loss.

CONDITIONS: for full yin blood diseases.

Fu ling yin
Bukukyoin

5 ch'ien	fu ling
4	ts'ang chu
3	jen shen
3	ch'ên p'i
3	shêng chiang
1.5	chih shih

PROPERTIES: carminative; stomachic.

CONDITIONS: to be used for approximately one week and no longer.

---

*This tea is made from a fine powder purchased ready-made from traditional pharmaceutical firms. It contains a great many herbs, none of which is uncommon. The preparation of the herbs, the grinding and mixing, is a very tedious procedure. Since it is impractical to prepare this tea on an individual basis, the recipe is not included here.

Fu tzu t'ang
  Bushito

5 ch'ien	fu ling
4	shao yao
4	ts'ang chu
3	jen shen
0.5	fu tzu

半夏湯

茯苓 五夏
芍藥 四夏
朮 四夏
人参 三夏
半夏 半夏

PROPERTIES: antidiarrhetic; antidiuretic; tonic.

CONDITIONS: for very yin people only.

Hsi kan ming mu t'ang
  Senkanmeimokuto

1.5 ch'ien	tang kuei
1.5	hsiung ch'iung
1.5	shao yao
1.5	ti huang
1.5	huang ch'in
1.5	chih tzû mien
1.5	lien ch'iao
1.5	fang feng
1.5	chüeh ming tzu
1.5	huang lien
1.5	ching chieh
1.5	p'u ho
1.5	chiang huo
1.5	man ching tzu
1.5	chü hua
1.5	chieh keng
1.5	chi li tzu
1.5	kan ts'ao
3	shih kao

洗肝明目湯

當歸 一夏半
川芎 一夏半
芍藥 一夏半
地黃 一夏半
黃芩 一夏半
山梔子 一夏半
連翹 一夏半

防風 一夏半
決明子 一夏半
黃連 一夏半
荊芥 一夏半
薄荷 一夏半
羌活 一夏半

蔓荊子 二夏
菊花 一夏半
桔梗 一夏半
蒺藜子 一夏半
甘草 一夏半
石膏 一夏半

PROPERTIES: cooling; benefits the liver; treats eye disorders related to
  liver disorders.

Hsiang su t'ang
Kososan

香蘇散

4 ch'ien	hsiang fu tzu
1	su yeh
2.5	ch'ên p'i
3	shêng chiang
1	kan ts'ao

甘草 生姜 陳皮 蘇葉 香附子

PROPERTIES: diaphoretic; vasotonic; treats common cold; treats insufficient menstruation or complete lack of menstruation; treats fish poisoning; treats mental disorders.

Hsiao ch'ai hu t'ang
Shosaikoto

小紫胡湯

7 ch'ien	ch'ai hu
5	pan hsia
4	shêng chiang
3	huang ch'in
3	tsao
3	jen shen
2	kan ts'ao

甘草 人参 大棗 黄芩 生姜 半夏 紫胡

PROPERTIES: tonic; stomachic; antiemetic; mild antipyretic; relieves fever accompanied by chills; treats small yang stage illness; treats common cold and influenza; treats bronchitis and tuberculosis; treats hepatitis; treats stomach and intestinal disorders.

CONDITIONS: for yin people; long usage recommended. May be used for one to two years.

Hsiao ch'eng ch'i t'ang
Shojokito

小承気湯

3 ch'ien	hou p'o
2	chih shih
2	ta huang

大黄 枳實 厚朴

PROPERTIES: laxative; hypotensive; reduces obesity; treats mental disorders attributed to hypertension; treats food poisoning.

CONDITIONS: for yang people; to be taken for a short time only, one week at most.

Hsiao chien chung t'ang
  Shokenchuto

4 ch'ien	kuei
4	shêng chiang
4	tsao
6	shao yao
2	kan ts'ao
20	a chiao

PROPERTIES: tonic; relieves fatigue; reduces excessive urination; treats bed-wetting, wet dreaming, and night sweating.

CONDITIONS: for yin people and children of any type.

Hsiao ch'ing lung t'ang
  Shoseiryuto

3 ch'ien	ma huang
3	shao yao
3	kan chiang
3	kan ts'ao
3	kuei
3	hsi hsin
3	wu wei tzu
6	pan hsia

PROPERTIES: expectorant; cooling; treats coughs, colds, bronchitis, asthma, and pneumonia; treats joint disorders; treats kidney disorders.

CONDITIONS: for yang people; use for a short time only.

Hsiao pan hsia fu ling t'ang
  Shohangebukuryototo

6 ch'ien	pan hsia
6	chiang
5	fu ling

PROPERTIES: antiemetic; treats morning sickness.

CONDITIONS: for yang people.

Hsing ch'uan chieh tu t'ang
Kangawagedokuto

4 ch'ien	t'u fu ling
4	mu t'ung
5	fu ling
3	hsiung ch'iung
3	jen tung
1	kan ts'ao
1	ta huang

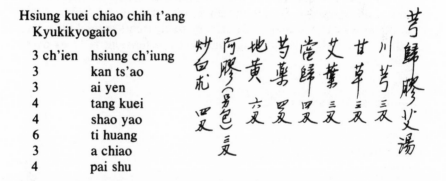

PROPERTIES: diuretic; treats syphilitic conditions.

CONDITIONS: requires extended usage.

Hsiung kuei chiao chih t'ang
Kyukikyogaito

3 ch'ien	hsiung ch'iung
3	kan ts'ao
3	ai yen
4	tang kuei
4	shao yao
6	ti huang
3	a chiao
4	pai shu

PROPERTIES: hemocathartic; hemostatic; treats anemia; treats hemorrhoids; treats intestinal and uterine bleeding.

Huang chü chien chung t'ang
Ohgikenchuto

4 ch'ien	huang ch'i
4	kuei
4	shêng chiang
4	tsao
6	shao yao
2	kan ts'ao
20	chiao i

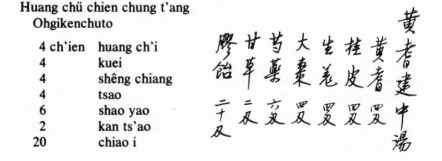

PROPERTIES: tonic; treats bed-wetting and night crying; treats pneumonia and asthma; treats stomach-ache; treats eye hemorrhages.

Huang lien chieh tu t'ang
Ohrengedokuto

1.5 ch'ien	huang lien
3	huang ch'in
1.5	huang po
2	chih tzû mien

PROPERTIES: cooling; hypotensive; anti-inflammatory and hemostatic; used to treat hemorrhagic conditions such as blood raising, bloody urine, and epistaxis; treats cerebral hemorrhage and hemorrhagic conditions of the stomach and urinary tract; treats mental disorders related to cerebral hemorrhage and/or hypertension; reduces over-excitability.

CONDITIONS: for yang people.

Huang tu t'ang
Ohdoto

7 ch'ien	huang tu
3	ti huang
3	ts'ang chu
3	a chiao
3	huang ch'in
2	kan ts'ao
0.5	fu tzu

PROPERTIES: warming; coagulant and hemostatic; used to treat hemorrhagic conditions such as blood raising, blood evacuation, bloody stool, bloody urine, and epistaxis; treats hemorrhagic conditions of the stomach, intestines, anus, kidneys, bladder, and uterus; treats anemia; relieves cold hands and feet.

Jun ch'ang t'ang
  Junchyoto

3 ch'ien	tang kuei
3	shu ti huang
3	kan ti huang
2	ma jen
2	t'ao jen
2	hsing jen
2	chih ka
2	hou p'o
2	huang ch'in
2	ta huang
1.5	kan ts'ao

潤腸湯

當歸 三叉

熟地黃 三叉

乾地黃 三叉

麻子仁 三叉

桃仁 三叉

杏仁 三叉

枳壳 二叉

厚朴 二叉

黃芩 二叉

大黃 二叉

甘草 一叉半

PROPERTIES: mild laxative.

CONDITIONS: for yin people and old people.

Kan mai ta tsao t'ang
  Kanbakudaisoto

5 ch'ien	kan ts'ao
6	tsao
20	hsiao mai (wheat)

甘麥大棗湯

甘草 五叉

大棗 六叉

小麥 二十叉

PROPERTIES: relaxant; mild sedative; relieves hysteria in women and children.

Kan ts'ao fu tzu t'ang
  Kanzobushito

2 ch'ien	kan ts'ao
4	ts'ang chu
3.5	kuei
0.5	fu tzu

甘草附子湯

甘草 二叉

尤草 三叉

桂枝 三叉半

附子 半叉

PROPERTIES: diuretic; treats arthritis, rheumatism, and general discomfort in the joints; treats gout.

CONDITIONS: for yin people.

88

Ke ken t'ang
Kakonto

8 ch'ien	ke ken
4	ma huang
4	shêng chiang
4	tsao
3	kuei
3	shao yao
2	kan ts'ao

甘 芍 桂 大 生 麻 葛
草 藥 枝 棗 薑 黃 根

PROPERTIES: strengthens the intestines, heart, liver, and kidneys; relieves headaches, colds, and stiff shoulders.

Kua lou chih shih t'ang
Karokijutsuto

3 ch'ien	tang kuei
3	fu ling
3	pei mu
2	kua lou shih
2	chieh keng
2	ch'ên p'i
2	huang chin
2	shêng chiang
1	so sha
1	ming cha
1	kan ts'ao
1	chih tzû mien
1	chih shih
1	chu ku

黃 陳 桔 瓜 貝 茯 當
芩 皮 梗 呂 母 苓 歸
　　　　實

竹 枳 梔 甘 木 縮 生
茹 實 子 草 香 砂 薑

PROPERTIES: expectorant; relieves coughs; treats bronchitis, asthma, and tuberculosis; treats heart attacks; treats acid indigestion.

Kua lou t'ang
Karoto

3 ch'ien	kua lou shih
6	pan hsia
4	hsieh pai
2	chih shih
2	shêng chiang

生 枳 薤 半 瓜
薑 實 白 夏 呂
　　　　實

PROPERTIES: cardiac stimulant; produces a strong, steady pulse; treats heart attacks and other heart disorders.

Kuei chiang tsao ts'ao hsin fu t'ang
Keikyososoohshinbuto

3 ch'ien	kuei	
3	shêng chiang	
3	tsao	
2	kan ts'ao	
2	ma huang	
2	hsi hsin	
0.5	fu tzu	

桂薑棗草黃辛附湯

PROPERTIES: promotes respiratory harmony; treats chronic conditions of combined yin chi and yang chi, such as bronchitis, asthma, recurring colds, arthritis, rheumatism, tuberculosis, paralysis, and swelling of the body.

CONDITIONS: for old men and weak people.

Kuei chih chia lung ku mu li t'ang
Keishikaryukotsuboreito

4 ch'ien	kuei	
4	shao yao	
4	tsao	
4	shêng chiang	
2	kan ts'ao	
2.5	lung ku	
2.5	mu li	

桂枝加龍骨牡蠣湯

PROPERTIES: tonic; vasotonic; relieves chills; sedative; treats wet dreaming and bed-wetting.

CONDITIONS: for weak people who tire quickly and are often and easily excited.

Kuei chih chia shao yao t'ang
Keishikashakuyakuto

4 ch'ien	kuei	
4	shêng chiang	
4	tsao	
2	kan ts'ao	
6	shao yao	

桂枝加芍藥湯

PROPERTIES: tonic; vasotonic; relieves chills, neuralgia, and headaches.

CONDITIONS: for yin people.

Kuei chih fu ling wan
Keishibukuryogan

3 ch'ien	kuei
3	fu ling
3	shao yao
3	mu tan pi
3	t'ao jen

桃仁　牡丹皮　芍藥　茯苓　桔枝　桂枝茯苓丸
羑　羑　羑　羑　羑

PROPERTIES: hemocathartic; clears the complexion; treats hemorrhoids; tonifies ovaries and uterus; spayolytic; treats frigidity and sterility; eases delivery during childbirth.

CONDITIONS: to ease delivery during childbirth, the tea should be employed by women whose bodies are either excessively yin or excessively yang. For other purposes, anyone may use this tea.

Kuei chih t'ang
Keishito

4 ch'ien	kuei
4	shao yao
4	tsao
4	shêng chiang
2	kan ts'ao

甘草　生羌　大棗　芍藥　桂枝　桂枝湯
二　四　四　四　四

PROPERTIES: tonic; vasotonic; relieves chills.

Kuei p'i t'ang
Kihito

2 ch'ien	huang ch'i
3	jen shen
3	ts'ang chu
3	fu ling
3	suan tsao jen
3	lung yen jou
2	tang kuei
1.5	shêng chiang
1.5	tsao
1.5	yüan chih
1	kan ts'ao
1	mu hsiang

歸脾湯
龍眼肉　酸棗仁　茯苓　朮　人參　黃耆
大香　甘草　遠志　大棗　生羌　當歸

PROPERTIES: stomachic; hematinic employed against anemia, leukemia, and hemophilia; hemostatic used for hemorrhagic conditions such as blood evacuation and blood raising; treats bleeding ulcers of the stomach and/or intestines, uterine bleeding, etc.; promotes a strong, steady heartbeat; treats certain mental disorders such as forgetfulness, insomnia, and wet dreaming; rejuvenative tonic.

CONDITIONS: for yin people.

Li chung t'ang
  Richuto

3 ch'ien	jen shen
3	kan ts'ao
3	ts'ang chu
3	kan chiang

PROPERTIES: tonic; strengthens the digestive system, particularly the stomach; tonifies the heart and circulatory system; treats anemia; improves sexual vitality.

CONDITIONS: for yin people.

Li hsiao san
  Rikkosan

2 ch'ien	hsi hsin
2	sheng ma
2	fang feng
1.5	kan ts'ao
1	lung tan tsao

PROPERTIES: hemocathartic; vasotonic; treats disorders of the teeth and gums; treats hemorrhoids.

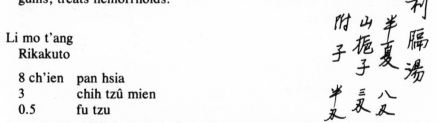

Li mo t'ang
  Rikakuto

8 ch'ien	pan hsia
3	chih tzû mien
0.5	fu tzu

PROPERTIES: warming; treats stomach disorders and stomach cancer; treats throat disorders and throat cancer.

CONDITIONS: for yin people.

Lien chu t'ang
  Renjuin

2 ch'ien	tang kuei
2	shao yao
2	hsiung ch'iung
2	ti huang
5	fu ling
3	kuei
2	ts'ang chu
2	kan ts'ao

甘草　尤　桂皮　茯苓　地黄　川芎　芍薬　当帰飲

連珠飲

PROPERTIES: hematinic; strengthens the intestines; vermicide.

Ling kan chiang wei hsin hsia jen t'ang
  Ryokankyoninshingeninto

4 ch'ien	fu ling
4	pan hsia
4	hsing jen
3	wu wei tzu
2	kan ts'ao
2	kan chiang
2	hsi hsin

細辛　乾姜　甘草　五味子　杏仁　半夏　茯苓

苓甘姜味辛夏仁湯

PROPERTIES: warming; diuretic; antitussive; treats coughs, asthma, bronchitis, and tuberculosis; treats heart valve disorders; treats stomach disorders; treats anemia; reduces fever and relieves fever accompanied by chills.

Ling kuei shu kan t'ang
  Ryokeijutsukanto

6 ch'ien	fu ling
4	kuei
3	ts'ang chu
2	kan ts'ao

甘草　尤　桂皮　茯苓

苓桂尤甘湯

PROPERTIES: diuretic; treats water disease; regulates the heartbeat; relieves dizziness; treats near- or farsightedness and general weak vision.

Lung tan hsieh kan t'ang
Ryutanshakanto

3 ch'ien	ch'e ch'ien tzu
3	huang chin
3	tsê hsieh
3	mu tung
3	ti huang
3	tang kuei
1.5	chih tzû mien
1.5	kan ts'ao
1.5	lung tan tsao

龍胆瀉肝湯
車前子 三戔
黃芩 三戔
澤瀉 三戔
木通 三戔
地黃 三戔
當歸 三戔
梔子 一戔半
甘草 一戔半
龍胆 一戔半

PROPERTIES: cooling; diuretic; syphilitic; treats sexual disorders including gonorrhea, syphillis, amoebic infections, leucorrhea, etc.; promotes a quick discharge from the sexual organs.

CONDITIONS: for yang people.

Ma hsing kan shih t'ang
Makyokansekito

4 ch'ien	ma huang
4	hsing jen
2	kan ts'ao
10	shih kao

麻杏甘石湯
麻黃 四戔
杏仁 四戔
甘草 二戔
石膏 十戔

PROPERTIES: cooling; antipyretic; analgesic; expectorant; antisudorific; treats children's colds; treats asthma.

Ma hsing yi kan t'ang
Makyoyokkonto

4 ch'ien	ma huang
3	hsing jen
10	i i jên
2	kan ts'ao

麻杏薏甘湯
麻黃 四戔
杏仁 三戔
薏苡仁 十戔
甘草 二戔

PROPERTIES: diuretic; treats water disease; treats skin disease and clears pimples, warts, and rashes; treats joint disorders; treats rheumatism.

Ma huang fu tzu hsi hsin t'ang
Maobushisaishinto

4 ch'ien	ma huang
3	hsi hsin
0.5	fu tzu

麻黄附子細辛湯

麻黄 三戋
細辛 三戋
附子 半戋

PROPERTIES: warming; tonic; treats colds; treats asthma and bronchitis; treats low fever; treats weak pulse; treats general weakness.

CONDITIONS: for yin people.

Ma huang t'ang
Maoto

5 ch'ien	ma huang
5	hsing jen
4	kuei
1.5	kan ts'ao

麻黄湯

麻黄 五戋
杏仁 五戋
桂枝 四戋
甘草 一戋半

PROPERTIES: diuretic; expectorant; suppresses appetite; promotes mental alertness; sometimes prevents sleep; treats colds, asthma, and congestion.

Ma tzu jen wan
Mashiningan

5 ch'ien	ma jen
2	shao yao
2	chih shih
2	hou p'o
2	ta huang
2	hsing jen

麻子仁丸

麻子仁 六戋
芍藥 二戋
枳實 二戋
厚朴 二戋
大黄 二戋
杏仁 二戋

PROPERTIES: mild laxative.

CONDITIONS: for yin people.

Mai men tung t'ang
Bakumondoto

10 ch'ien	mai men tung
5	pan hsia
5	keng mi
3	tsao
2	jen shen
2	kan ts'ao

麥門冬湯

麥門冬 十戋
半夏 五戋
粳米 五戋
大棗 三戋
人參 二戋
甘草 二戋

PROPERTIES: tonic; expectorant; treats coughs, bronchitis, and tuberculosis.

CONDITIONS: for yin people; may be taken for approximately one month.

Mu fang i t'ang
Mokuboito

4 ch'ien	mu fang
10	shih kao
3	kuei
3	jen shen

木防己湯
木防己　三罂
石膏　十支
桂皮　三支
人參　三支

PROPERTIES: diuretic; cardiac stimulant; promotes a strong and slow heartbeat; treats certain heart disorders; reduces swelling of the body due to heart disorders; treats asthma.

Pa wei wan
Hachimigan

6 ch'ien	ti huang
3	shan yao
3	shan chu yü
3	tsê hsieh
3	fu ling
3	mu tan pi
1	kuei
0.5	fu tzu

八味丸
地黄　六支
山藥　三支
山茱萸　三支
澤瀉　三支
茯苓　三支
牡丹皮　三支
桂枝　一支
附子　半支

PROPERTIES: tonic; induces harmony in the urinary tract; reduces excessive urination and encourages urination when there is too little; tonifies weak kidneys and sexual organs; treats eye conditions related to weak kidneys.

CONDITIONS: for weak people, small ying people, and especially old people who are yin.

Pai hu chia jen shen t'ang
Byakkoto

White tiger tea

5 ch'ien	chih mu
8	keng mi (rice)
15	shih kao
2	kan ts'ao
2	jen shen

白虎加人參湯
知母　五支
粳米　八支
石膏　十五支
甘草　二支
人參　三支

PROPERTIES: induces harmony; antipyretic; analgesic; abates thirst.

CONDITIONS: may be used for approximately two to three months.

Pan hsia hou p'o t'ang
  Hangekobokuto

6 ch'ien	pan hsia
6	fu ling
4	chiang
3	hou p'o
2	su yeh

蘇葉 厚朴 生姜 茯苓 半夏 半夏厚朴湯

二叉 三叉 罒叉 六叉 六叉

PROPERTIES: treats chi diseases, especially mental disorders; antiemetic; treats morning sickness.

CONDITIONS: for yang people.

Pan hsia hsieh hsin t'ang
  Hangeshashinto

5 ch'ien	pan hsia
2.5	huang ch'in
2.5	kan chiang
2.5	jen shen
2.5	kan ts'ao
2.5	tsao
1	huang lien

黄連 大棗 甘草 人參 乾姜 黄芩 半夏 半夏瀉心湯

一叉 二叉半 二叉半 二叉半 二叉半 二叉半 五叉

PROPERTIES: antiemetic; antidiarrhetic; stomachic.

P'ing wei san
  Heisan

4 ch'ien	ts'ang chu
3	hou p'o
3	ch'ên p'i
2	shêng chiang
2	tsao
1	kan ts'ao

甘草 大棗 生姜 陳皮 厚朴 蒼朮 平胃散

一叉 三叉 二叉 三叉 三叉 罒叉

PROPERTIES: stomachic; treats acid indigestion and ulcers.

CONDITIONS: for yang people only. This tea is employed before any other in the treatment of hypochondriac patients whose descriptions of their stomach ailments are so excessive as to render clear diagnosis impossible.

Pu chung yi ch'i t'ang
Hochuekkito

4 ch'ien	huang ch'i
4	jen shen
4	ts'ang chu
3	tang kuei
2	ch'ên p'i
2	shêng chiang
2	tsao
2	ch'ai hu
1.5	kan ts'ao
1	sheng ma

PROPERTIES: tonic; diuretic.

CONDITIONS: for yin people.

P'u kung ying t'ang
Hokoeito

8 ch'ien	p'u kung ying
6	tang kuei
3	hsiang fu tzu
3	mu tan pi
4	shan yao

PROPERTIES: lactogogue; stomachic; vasotonic.

San huang hsieh hsin t'ang
Sanohshashinto

1 ch'ien	huang lien
1	huang ch'in
1	ta huang

PROPERTIES: cooling; hypotensive; treats certain mental disorders attri-

98

buted to hypertension such as overexcitability; coagulant; treats epistaxis and bleeding from the stomach wall.

CONDITIONS: for yang people.

San wei che ku ts'ai t'ang
Sanmishakosaito

5 ch'ien	che ku ts'ai
2	kan ts'ao
2	ta huang

三味鷹胡菜湯

大黃　甘草　鷹胡菜
三灵　三灵　五灵

PROPERTIES: vermicide; treats overeating, abdominal pain, and malnutrition; treats anemia.

Shao kan huang hsin fu t'ang
Shakukanohshinbuto

3 ch'ien	shao yao
3	kan ts'ao
2	hsi hsin
1	ta huang
0.5	fu tzu

芍甘黃辛附湯

附子　大黃　細辛　甘草　芍藥
半灵　一灵　二灵　三灵　三灵

PROPERTIES: warming; analgesic; hemocathartic; treats arthritis, rheumatism, and binding of the spine.

CONDITIONS: not suitable for very yang people. The amount of fu tzu should be increased .1 ch'ien each week that the tea is used, starting with .3 ch'ien and holding at .5 ch'ien if treatment continues beyond three weeks.

芍藥甘草湯

甘草　芍藥
五灵　五灵

Shao yao kan ts'ao t'ang
Shakuyakukanzoto

| 5 ch'ien | shao yao |
| 5 | kan ts'ao |

PROPERTIES: analgesic; relieves any sharp abdominal pain such as pain caused by gallstones, kidney stones, stomach cramps, etc.

Shih ch'uan ta pu t'ang
  Jujendaihoto

3 ch'ien	jen shen
3	huang ch'i
4	ts'ang chu
4	tang kuei
4	fu ling
4	ti huang
3	hsiung ch'iung
3	shao yao
3	kuei
2	kan ts'ao

PROPERTIES: tonic; hematopoietic; treats scrofula.

CONDITIONS: for yin people.

Shih shen ming mu t'ang
  Jijinmeimokuto

3 ch'ien	tang kuei
3	hsiung chiung
3	ti huang
3	shu ti huang
3	shao yao
1.5	chieh keng
1.5	chih tzû mien
1.5	jen shen
1.5	huang lien
1.5	pai chih
1.5	man ching tzu
1.5	chü hua
1.5	kan ts'ao
1.5	teng hsin ts'ao
1.5	hsi cha

PROPERTIES: regulates urination; relieves eye disorders resulting from kidney malfunction; relieves vitamin B complex deficiency; promotes the growth of beneficial intestinal flora.

CONDITIONS: for yin people. May be used for approximately two to three months.

100

Shih wei t'iao tu t'ang
Jumihaidokuto

3 ch'ien	ch'ai hu
3	ying pi
3	chieh keng
3	shêng chiang
3	hsiung ch'iung
3	fu ling
2	tu huo
2	fang feng
2	kan ts'ao
2	ching chieh

十味排毒湯

紫胡　櫻皮　桔梗　生姜　川芎　茯苓　獨活　防瓜　甘草　荊芥
三　三　三　三　三　三　三　三　三　三

PROPERTIES: diuretic; treats yang kidney disorders, insufficient urination, and skin ulcers and rashes which result from this condition; treats syphilis.

CONDITIONS: for yang people.

Su tzu chiang ch'i t'ang
Soshikokito

3 ch'ien	su tzu
4	pan hsia
2.5	ch'ên p'i
2.5	hou p'o
2.5	ch'ien hu
2.5	kuei
2.5	tang kuei
1.5	tsao
1.5	shêng chiang
1	kan ts'ao

蘇子降氣湯

蘇子　半夏　陳皮　厚朴　前胡
三　四　二半　二半　二半
桂枝　當歸　大棗　生姜　甘草
二半　二半　一半　一半　一

PROPERTIES: treats chi diseases; removes excess chi from the head; relieves cold feet; reduces excess mucus in the throat and eases breathing; treats bronchitis; treats hemoptysis, epistaxis, and bleeding gums.

Suan tsao jen t'ang
Sansoninto

甘　茯　川　知　酸　酸
草　苓　芎　母　棗　棗
　　　　　　仁　仁
　　　　　　　　湯
一　一　三　三　十
又　又　又　又　又

PROPERTIES: tonic; benefits the nervous system; analgesic; treats both insomnia and excessive sleeping.

CONDITIONS: for yin people.

Szu chün tzu t'ang
Shikunshito

大　生　甘　茯　尢　人　四
棗　姜　草　苓　　　參　君
　　　　　　　　　　　子
　　　　　　　　　　　湯
一　一　一　四　罗　罗
又　又　又　又　又　又
半　半　半

PROPERTIES: tonic; stomachic; antiemetic; antidiarrhetic; treats stomach and intestinal disorders including bleeding along the digestive tract; treats bed-wetting; treats anemia; sometimes used to treat paralysis.

CONDITIONS: though anyone may use it, this tea is especially effective for yin people.

Szu ni t'ang
Shigyakuto

桂　附　乾　甘　四
枝　子　姜　草　逆
　　　　　　　湯
三　半　二　三
又　又　又　又

PROPERTIES: tonic; warming; stimulates the metabolism; antidiarrhetic; relieves cold hands and feet; brings color to the face; relieves stomach-aches.

CONDITIONS: for yin people.

Szu ti t'ang
Shiteito

5 ch'ien	szu ti
1.5	ting hsiang
4	shêng chiang

PROPERTIES: spasmolytic; relieves hiccups.

柿蒂湯
生薑 丁香 柿蒂
五戈 一戈半

Szu wu t'ang
Shimotsuto

4 ch'ien	tang kuei
4	shao yao
4	ti huang
4	hsiung ch'iung

PROPERTIES: hemotopoietic; hemocathartic; vasotonic; spasmolytic; analgesic; treats gynecopathy, especially menstrual disorders and vaginal infections; treats anemia; beautifies the skin.

四物湯
川芎 地黄 芍藥 當歸

Ta ch'ai hu chia lung ku mu li t'ang
Daisaikokaryukotsuboreito

6 ch'ien	ch'ai hu
4	pan hsia
4	shêng chiang
3	huang ch'in
3	shao yao
3	tsao
2	chih shih
1	ta huang
3	lung ku
3	mu li

大柴胡加龍骨牡蠣湯

PROPERTIES: laxative; hypotensive; treats gall bladder disorders, especially gallstones; treats stomach disorders; treats asthma and coughs; reduces obesity; benefits the nervous system; treats mental disorders attributed to hypertension.

CONDITIONS: for extremely yang people; may be used for approximately one month.

Ta ch'ai hu t'ang
Daisaikoto

6 ch'ien	ch'ai hu
4	pan hsia
4	shêng chiang
3	huang ch'in
3	shao yao
3	tsao
2	chih shih
1	ta huang

大柴胡湯
柴胡 六戔
半夏 四戔
生姜 四戔
黄芩 三戔
芍藥 三戔
大棗 三戔
枳實 二戔
大黄 一戔

PROPERTIES: laxative; hypotensive; treats gall bladder disorders, especially gallstones; treats stomach disorders; treats asthma and coughs; reduces obesity.

CONDITIONS: for extremely yang people; may be used for approximately one month.

Ta ch'eng ch'i t'ang
Daijokito

2 ch'ien	ta huang
3	chih shih
3	mang hsiao
5	hou p'o

大承氣湯
大黄 二戔
枳實 三戔
芒硝 三戔
厚朴 五戔

PROPERTIES: strong laxative; vasotonic; disperses bruises; reduces bleeding from internal hemorrhages; treats both excessive and insufficient menstrual flow and relieves mental disorders (such as depression) which result from menstrual disorders; disperses certain types of uterine tumors; promotes the discharge of afterbirth; relieves certain skin diseases.

CONDITIONS: for yang people; use for a short time.

Ta ch'ing lung t'ang
Daiseiryuto

6 ch'ien	ma huang
5	hsing jen
3	kuei
3	shêng chiang
3	tsao
2	kan ts'ao
10	shih kao

大青龍湯
麻黄 六戔
杏仁 五戔
桂枝 三戔
生姜 三戔
大棗 三戔
甘草 二戔
石膏 十戔

PROPERTIES: expectorant; cooling; treats colds, fevers, influenza, and pneumonia; treats joint and muscle pain, especially in the area of the buttocks.

Ta huang fu tzu t'ang
Diaobushito

1 ch'ien	ta huang
0.5	fu tzu
2	hsi hsin

PROPERTIES: laxative; warming; abdominal relaxant; treats gout and similar ailments.

CONDITIONS: for yin people.

Ta huang mu tan t'ang
Daiobotanpito

2 ch'ien	ta huang
4	mu tan pi
4	t'ao jen
4	mang hsiao
6	kua tzu

PROPERTIES: vasotonic; laxative; relieves chronic conditions of the lower abdomen such as hemorrhoids, gonorrhea, chronic appendicitis, and similar yang conditions of the intestines, uterus, ovaries, anus, bladder, and urinary tract.

CONDITIONS: for yang people and yang blood disease.

Tang kuei chien chung t'ang
Tokikenchuto

4 ch'ien	tang kuei
4	kuei
4	shêng chiang
4	tsao
5	shao yao
2	kan ts'ao

PROPERTIES: warming; relieves lower abdomen pain; treats uterine bleeding and menstrual disorders; treats arthritis.

Tang kuei szu ni chia wu chu yü shêng chiang t'ang
Tokishigyakukagoshuyukyoto

3 ch'ien	tang kuei
3	kuei
3	shao yao
3	mu tung
2	hsi hsin
2	kan ts'ao
5	tsao
2	wu chu yü
4	shêng chiang

PROPERTIES: tonic; strengthens the nervous and glandular systems; promotes sexual vitality; stimulates circulation, especially in the hands, feet, and pelvic region; increases the sensitivity of women's sexual organs.

CONDITIONS: for yin people.

Tang kuei t'iao yao san
Tokishakuyakusan

3 ch'ien	tang kuei
3	hsiung ch'iung
4	shao yao
4	fu ling
4	ts'ang chu
4	tsê hsieh

PROPERTIES: hemocathartic; clears the complexion; treats hemorrhoids; tonifies the ovaries and uterus; relieves cramps; treats frigidity and sterility; eases delivery at childbirth.

CONDITIONS: generally for somewhat yin people. To ease delivery at childbirth, however, women with more balanced bodies should use this tea rather than kuei chih fu ling wan.

Ti tang wan
Teitogan

1 ch'ien	shui chih
1	mang ch'ung
1	t'ao jen
3	ta huang

PROPERTIES: anticoagulant; hemocathartic; vasotonic; "melts" blood clots and prevents clotting of internal hemorrhages when clotting is not desirable, as in some cases of concussion, etc.; treats mental disorders arising from blood clots on the brain; treats interrupted menstrual flow, uterine tumors, and related conditions; treats yang blood disease, making the blood more yin.

CONDITIONS: for yang people.

T'iao wei ch'eng ch'i t'ang
Choijokito

2 ch'ien	ta huang
1	mang hsiao
1	kan ts'ao

調胃承氣湯

甘草 芒硝 大黄

灸 一兩 二兩

PROPERTIES: laxative; hypotensive; reduces obesity; treats certain mental disorders attributed to hypotension; treats food poisoning.

CONDITIONS: for yang people; to be taken for a short time only, one week at most.

Ts'ao ho ch'eng ch'i t'ang
Tokakujokito

5 ch'ien	t'ao jen
4	kuei
2	mang hsiao
3	ta huang
1.5	kan ts'ao

桃核承氣湯

甘草 大黄 芒硝 桂枝 桃核仁

灸半 三兩 二兩 四兩 五兩

PROPERTIES: strong laxative; vasotonic; disperses bruises; reduces bleeding from internal hemorrhages; treats both excessive and insufficient menstrual flow and relieves mental disorders (such as depression) which result from menstrual disorders; disperses certain types of uterine tumors; promotes the discharge of afterbirth; relieves certain skin diseases.

CONDITIONS: for yang people; use for a short time.

T'ung tao san
Tsudosanshazenshi

3 ch'ien	ta huang
3	chih shih
3	tang kuei
3	mang hsiao
2	hou p'o
2	ch'ên p'i
2	mu tung
2	hung hua
2	su mu
2	kan ts'ao

PROPERTIES: vasotonic; hemocathartic.

CONDITIONS: for yang people. This tea is similar to ts'ao ho ch'eng ch'i t'ang but not quite so strong; it may therefore be used more widely.

Wei cheng fang
Ishoho

4 ch'ien	tang kuei
4	ti huang
3	ts'ang chu
3	niu hsi
3	chih mu
3	shao yao
3	huang ch'i
2	tu chung
2	huang po

PROPERTIES: vasotonic; osteogenic; treats weakness, paralysis, or numbness of the limbs, especially the legs; improves kidney function and speeds removal of excess fluid; strengthens muscles that have been weakened by polio or paralysis.

CONDITIONS: for yang people.

Wen ch'ing yin
Unsei-in

温清飲

4 ch'ien	tang kuei
4	ti huang
3	shao yao
3	hsiung ch'iung
3	huang ch'in
2	chih tzû mien
1.5	huang lien
1.5	huang po

黄柏 黄連 栀子 黄芩 川芎 芍藥 地黄 當歸

一半 一半 二戋 三戋 三戋 三戋 四戋 四戋

PROPERTIES: vasotonic; coagulant; hypotensive; treats itchy skin diseases and allergic skin reactions; treats liver disorders; promotes harmony in the autonomic nervous system.

CONDITIONS: this is at once both a yin and a yang tea.

Wu chi san
Goshakusan

五積散

4 ch'ien	ts'ang chu
2	ch'ên p'i
2	fu ling
2	pan hsia
2	tang kuei
1	hou p'o
1	shao yao
1	hsiung ch'iung
1	pai chih
1	chih shih
1	chieh keng
1	kan chiang
1	kuei
1	ma huang
1	chiang
1	kan ts'ao

川芎 芍藥 厚朴 當歸 半夏 茯苓 陳皮 尤

二戋 二戋 二戋 二戋 二戋 二戋 二戋 四戋

甘草 生姜 麻黄 桂皮 乾姜 桔梗 枳實 白芷

一戋 一戋 一戋 一戋 一戋 一戋 一戋 一戋

PROPERTIES: tonic; treats chi diseases; treats water disease and bladder disorders; vasotonic; treats anemia; treats illness attributed to cold and humidity; treats stomach disorders; relieves menstrual pain; treats pelvic disorders.

CONDITIONS: for yin people.

Wu ling t'ang
Goreisan

5 ch'ien	tsê hsieh
3	chu ling
3	fu ling
3	ts'ang chu
2	kuei

五苓散

桂枝 白朮 茯苓 猪苓 澤瀉

二爻 三爻 三爻 三爻 五爻

PROPERTIES: diuretic; treats kidney malfunctions and relieves swelling due to them; relieves swelling during pregnancy.

CONDITIONS: for yang people; to be used for a short time only.

Wu wei keng t'ang
Gosshuyuto

3 ch'ien	wu chu yü
2	jen shen
4	tsao
4	chiang

吳茱萸湯

生羗 大棗 人參 吳茱萸 吳茱萸

四爻 四爻 二爻 三爻

PROPERTIES: vasotonic; warming.

CONDITIONS: for yin people.

Yi kan san
Yokukansan

3 ch'ien	tang kuei
3	tiao têng kou
3	hsiung ch'iung
4	ts'ang chu
4	fu ling
2	ch'ai hu
1.5	kan ts'ao

抑肝散

甘草 柴胡 茯苓 朮 川芎 鈎藤 當歸

一爻半 三爻 三爻 四爻 四爻 三爻 三爻

PROPERTIES: cooling; diuretic; analgesic; treats liver disorders; treats children's fainting; treats mental and nervous system disorders such as hysteria, insomnia, gritting of the teeth during sleep, impotence, epilepsy, polio, and paralysis.

CONDITIONS: for yang people.

Yi tzu t'ang
  Otsujito

1 ch'ien	ta huang
5	ch'ai hu
1.5	sheng ma
2	kan ts'ao
3	huang ch'in
6	kuei

乙字湯

當歸　黃芩　甘草　升麻　柴胡　大黃

方又　三又　三又　一又半　五又　一又

PROPERTIES: warming; softens the feces; mild laxative; relieves bleeding and pain of hemorrhoids; relieves itching of the vagina; treats certain skin diseases and eruptions.

Yi yi jen t'ang
  Yokuinto

4 ch'ien	ma huang
4	tang kuei
4	ts'ang chu
8	i'i jên
3	kuei
3	shao yao
2	kan ts'ao

薏苡仁湯

甘草　芍藥　桂枝　薏苡仁　尤　當歸　麻黃

二又　三又　三又　八又　罢又　罢又　罢又

PROPERTIES: treats rheumatism and joint disorders and discomfort; treats vitamin B complex deficiency.

Yin ch'en kao t'ang
  Inchinkoto

4 ch'ien	yin ch'en
3	chih tzû mien
1	ta huang

茵陳蒿湯

大黃　茵陳　山梔子

一又　三又　罢又

PROPERTIES: treats liver and gall bladder disorders, especially jaundice; treats food poisoning.

CONDITIONS: for yang people; may be used for five to seven days.

Yin ch'en wu ling san
Inchingoreisan

4 ch'ien	yin ch'en
5	tsê hsieh
3	chu ling
3	fu ling
3	ts'ang chu
2	kuei

茵陳五苓散

桂枝 白朮 茯苓 豬苓 澤瀉 茵陳
二又 三又 三又 三又 五又 四又

PROPERTIES: diuretic; treats liver, gall bladder, and kidney disorders, i.e., jaundice, gallstones, insufficient urination, excessive thirst, and constipation.

CONDITIONS: for yang people; may be used for two weeks.

Yüeh pei t'ang
Eppito

6 ch'ien	ma huang
8	shih kao
3	chiang
3	tsao
2	kan ts'ao
4	ts'ang chu

越婢湯

朮 甘草 大棗 生薑 石膏 麻黃
四又 二又 三又 三又 八又 六又

PROPERTIES: diuretic; treats kidney conditions and swelling of the body.

Chapter 6
MOST COMMONLY USED CHINESE HERBS

(In Romanized Alphabetical Order with Annotated Chinese Characters)

Chinese medicinal herbs differ from Western herbs in that the former are not merely dried botanically but actually crude drugs which in some cases have been processed through several steps such as selection, cutting, peeling, scrubbing, leeching, roasting, and so on. These methods of preparation are often performed painstakingly by hand in a carefully prescribed manner that has been handed down from generation to generation since time immemorial. These methods of preparation are thought to alter considerably the quality of the basic material. Another dissimilarity lies in the fact that the Chinese herbs are rarely employed as individual agents. Most frequently they are used as building blocks in conjunction with other materials, so that the materials working in concert enhance or negate certain qualities of one another and produce a more effective pharmaceutical than the crude drugs alone. Occasionally some of these crude drugs are used in salves, liniments, plasters, or in other ways. Whenever this is the case it is indicated in the list below.

A chiao

   Akyo
   Equus Asinus
   Donkey

阿膠

The crude drug is donkey skin.

PROPERTIES: coagulant; tonic.

Ai yen

Gaiyo, Kaiyo
Artemisia princeps, A. vulgaris, A. capillaris
Mugwort, Wormwood

The crude drug is the leaves.

PROPERTIES: hematopoietic; antidiarrhetic; emmenagogue; diuretic; sudorific; vermicide; stomachic; treats asthma.

Ch'ai hu

Saiko
Bupleurum falcatum
Thorough wax

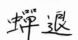

The crude drug is the dried stalks.

PROPERTIES: antipyretic; analgesic, especially for pain in head or chest; relieves nausea, anxieties, and dizziness; strengthens the eyes; strengthens the limbs—especially recommended for toning up leg muscles.

Ch'an t'uei, Ch'en t'uei, Shan t'uei

Zentai
Graptopsaltria nigrofuscata

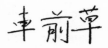

The crude drug is the dried shells of the cicada.

PROPERTIES: antipyretic.

Ch'e chi'en tsao

Shazensho
Plantago asiatica, P. major
Plantain

The crude drug is the whole dried plant.

PROPERTIES: diuretic; antitussive; increases sperm and fertility; antidiarrhetic; tonic; treats eye trouble; treats sexual disorders.

Ch'e chi'en tzu

    Shazenshi
    Plantago asiatica, P. major
    Plantain

車前子

The crude drug is the seeds.

PROPERTIES: diuretic; antitussive; increases sperm and fertility; antidiarrhetic; tonic; treats eye trouble; treats sexual disorders.

Che ku ts'ai

    Shakosai, Kaiso
    Digenea simplex

鷓鴣菜

The crude drug is the whole dried seaweed.

PROPERTIES: vermicide.

Ch'ên p'i

    Chinpi
    Citrus unshui, C. nobilis
    Orange peel

陳皮

The crude drug is the dried rind, older rinds being preferred because aging breaks down the bitter substances in the herb.

PROPERTIES: diuretic; antitussive; stomachic.

Ch'en t'uei (see Ch'an t'uei)

Chi li tzu

    Shitsurishi
    Ulex (species)
    Furze

蒺棃子

The crude drug is the berries.

PROPERTIES: tonic; treats weakness or afflictions of the eyes.

Chiang (see also Kan chiang and Shêng chiang)

    Kyo
    Zingiber officinale
    Ginger

生姜

The crude drug is the fresh rhizome.

PROPERTIES: stomachic; cardiac stimulant.

Chiang huo

Kyokatsu
Notoplerygium incisum

The crude drug is the rhizome.

PROPERTIES: diaphoretic; analgesic; antipyretic.

Chiao i, Kung mai nieh

Ko-i
Hordeium vulgare
Malted barley

The crude drug is the confection.

PROPERTIES: tonic.

Chieh keng

Kikyo
Platycodon grandiflorum
Balloon flower

The crude drug is the root.

PROPERTIES: antitussive; expectorant; antiphlogistic; relieves sore
throat, toothache, eye inflammation; treats hemorrhoids and skin
disease; treats dry coughs; carminative.

Ch'ien hu

Zenko
Peucedanum dicursivum

The crude drug is the root.

PROPERTIES: approximates ch'ai hu.

Chih ka

Kikoku
Citrus aurantium, C. nobilis
Sweet tangerine

The crude drug is the green skin of the fruit which has been dried.

PROPERTIES: expectorant; stomachic; constrictive; dries up running and itchy skin inflammations.

The bark of the roots is sometimes steeped in liquor to make a medicinal tincture. The bark of the roots is called chih k'o.

Chih kan tsao

Shakanzo
Glycyrrhiza glabra
Licorice

The crude drug is the root which has been dried and roasted.

PROPERTIES: cardiac stimulant.

Chih mu

Chimo
Anemarrhena asphodeloides

The crude drug is the rhizome.

PROPERTIES: sedative; antipyretic; diuretic; treats head colds accompanied by fever; treats gynecopathy.

Chih shih

Kyjitsu
Citrus aurantium, C. nobilis
Sweet tangerine

The crude drug is the green fruit which has been dried and roasted. This herb differs from chih ka in that it is gathered in a less mature state.

PROPERTIES: stomachic; expectorant.

Chih tzû mien

Sanshishi
Gardenia jasminoides

The crude drug is the ripe fruit.

PROPERTIES: encourages metabolism; diuretic; hemostatic.

The crude drug is used externally as a styptic, a treatment for skin diseases and traumas. The flowers are used in making jasmine tea.

Ching chieh

荊芥

Keigai
Schizonepeta tennuifolia

The crude drug is the seeds of the fruit.

PROPERTIES: diaphoretic; antipyretic; antitoxic; discharges poison.

Ching p'o po (see P'u kung ying)

Chü hua

菊花

Kikuka
Chrysanthemum moriflorium, C. sinense

The crude drug is the flowers.

PROPERTIES: antipyretic; antitoxic; analgesic; beneficial to the eyesight.

Chu ku, chu ju

竹茹

Chikujo
Puccinia corticoides
Bamboo leaves (species)

The crude drug is the leaves.

PROPERTIES: antipyretic; antitussive.

Chu ling

豬苓

Chorei
Grifola umbellata, Polyporus umbellatus

The crude drug is the mushroom.

PROPERTIES: diuretic; antipyretic; abates thirst.

Chü p'i

橘皮

Kippi
Citrus leiocarpa, C. nobilis
Orange peel

The crude drug is the dried peel. The older the peel the better, since aging allows for the breakdown of the bitter substances of the herb.

PROPERTIES: diuretic; antitussive; stomachic.

Ch'uan chiao, Shu chiao

Sanshyo
Zanthoxylum piperitum 川椒 蜀椒

The crude drug is the ripe fruit.

PROPERTIES: stomachic; vermicide; diuretic; spasmolytic.

Chuan hsiung (see Hsiung ch'iung)

Chüeh ming tzu

Habu
Cassia tora, Cassia obtusifolia, Cassia agustifolia
Foetid Cassia 決明子

The crude drug is the roasted seeds.

PROPERTIES: tonic; mild diuretic; mild laxative; improves eyesight.

Chung p'o po (see P'u kung ying)

Chung pu (see Hou p'o)

Fan hsieh yeh (see Chüeh ming tzu) 決明葉

Fang feng

Bofu
Ledebouriella seseloides 防風

The crude drug is the root.

PROPERTIES: sudorific; antipyretic; antitoxic; discharges poison.

Fu ling

Bukuryo
Pachyma cocos
Tuckahoe, Indian bread 茯苓

The crude drug is the mushroom sliced crosswise.

PROPERTIES: diuretic; stomachic; corrigent; aids in the circulation of drugs through the bloodstream.

Fu tzu

Bushi
Aconitum carmichaeli, A. fanriei, A. fisheri
Azure monkshood, Wolfbane

The crude drug is the root which has been dried, salted, and then roasted.

PROPERTIES: analgesic; diuretic; tonic; cardiac stimulant; treats rheumatism and neuralgia; antidiarrhetic; antipyretic; antitussive; treats smallpox, coughs, and colds.

The drug is extremely toxic. As little as a few grams may be lethal for a grown man. The alkaloids in this drug cause paralysis of the central nervous system; death follows by respiratory paralysis. This drug is not suitable for hypertensives.

Hou p'o, Chung pu

Koboku
Magnolia officinalis
Magnolia

The crude drug is the dried bark.

PROPERTIES: diuretic; expectorant; tonic; antiemetic; antidiarrhetic; analgesic for abdominal pain; improves vision.

Hsi cha

Saicha
Thea sinensis
Green tea

The crude drug is the leaves.

PROPERTIES: cardiac stimulant; diuretic; tonic.

Hsi hsin

Saishin
Asarum heterotropoides, A. Sieboldi
Wild ginger

The crude drug is rhizome and root.

PROPERTIES: analgesic; antitussive; expectorant; treats halitosis and aphtha; relieves congestion from head colds and blocked-up nose; treats watering eyes and hearing defects; diaphoretic.

Hsiang fu tzu

> Kobushi
> Cyperus rotundus

香附子

The crude drug is the root.

PROPERTIES: emmenagogue; analgesic, especially for headaches.

Hsiao mai

> Kanmi
> Triticum vulgare
> Wheat

小麦

The crude drug is the grain.

PROPERTIES: benefits the liver; nutrient; diuretic; demulcent; antihemorrhagic.

Hsieh pai

> Gaihaku
> Allium ascallonicum
> Scallion

薤白

The crude drug is the white bulb of the scallion.

PROPERTIES: cardiac stimulant.

Hsin i

> Shin-i
> Magnolia denudata

辛夷

The crude drug is the flower bud.

PROPERTIES: analgesic for headaches; discharges pus; demulcent.

Hsing jen

Kyonin
Prunus armeniaca
Apricot kernels

The crude drug is the kernel.

PROPERTIES: expectorant; antitussive; diuretic.

Hsiung ch'iung, Chuan hsiung

Senkyu
Ligusticum Wallichii, Cnidium officinale

The crude drug is the rhizome which has been dried after having been immersed in hot water.

PROPERTIES: vasotonic; analgesic, especially for headaches; sedative.

The best quality Hsiung ch'iung comes from Szechuan Province.

Hsuan fu hua

Senpukuka
Inula britannica
Elecampane

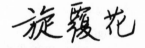

The crude drug is the dried flowers.

PROPERTIES: stomachic; expectorant; especially effective for deep-seated coughs; diuretic; vasotonic; reduces swelling due to intestinal dropsy; relieves neuralgia in head and eyes.

The crude drug is used to make a soothing salve for pulled muscles and fractures.

Hua shih

Kasseky
Collinite, Kasan aluminum

The crude drug is the mineral.

PROPERTIES: diuretic; abates thirst.

Huai hsiang

Uikyo
Foeniculum vulgare
Fennel

The crude drug is the fruit.

PROPERTIES: stomachic; carminative; analgesic; expectorant; treats eye catarrh; treats hernia.

Huai hua

Kaika
Sophora japonica
Pagoda tree

The crude drug is the flower bud.

PROPERTIES: analgesic; reduces blood pressure; styptic; hemostatic; used for hemorrhage conditions such as epistaxis, hemoptysis, and evacuation of blood from the bowels.

Huang ch'i

Ohgi
Astragalus mongholicus, A. membranaceus, A. hoantschy
Locoweed, Milk Vetch, Poison Vetch

The crude drug is the root.

PROPERTIES: diuretic; tonic; diaphoretic; hematinic; drains pus from boils; fortifies the triple warmer, spleen, and stomach.

Huang ch'in

Ohgon
Scutellaria baicalensis
Skull cap

The crude drug is the root.

PROPERTIES: diuretic; laxative; antipyretic; hemostatic; used to treat hemoptysis, bloody stool, and epistaxis; tonic; treats tuberculosis.

Huang hua, Hung lan hua

Koka
Carthamus tinctorius
Safflower

The crude drug is the dried corolla of the tubulous flower.

PROPERTIES: vasotonic; analgesic; hemotopoietic; emmenagogue.

The juice of the flower is germicidal.

Huang lien

Ohren
Coptis sinensis, C. japonica
Golden thread

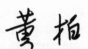

The crude drug is the rhizome.

PROPERTIES: stomachic; analgesic; antidiarrhetic; antipyretic; anti-inflammatory; relieves swellings of the face; relieves various types of congestion and hemorrhage.

In China genuine Huang lien is rare. It is often replaced with the Hu huang lien, the rhizome of Picorrhiza kurroa benth. The main active ingredients in this herb are alkaloids of the berberine group: berberine, palmatine, coptisine, and wozenine.

Huang po

Ohbaku
Phellodendron amurense
Yellow bark

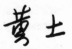

The crude drug is the bark with the cork layer removed.

PROPERTIES: stomachic; bactericide.

Because of this herb's bactericidal properties a decoction of it is often used as an eyewash.

Huang tu

Ohdo
Yellow clay

The crude drug is powdered yellow clay from an old earthen fireplace.

PROPERTIES: antiemetic; coagulant.

Huo ma (see Ma jen)

I i jên, Ma yuen

Yokuinin
Coix lacryma jobi
Job's tears

The crude drug is the ripe, hulled grains.

PROPERTIES: pus clearing; anti-inflammatory; vasotonic; analgesic; diuretic; purgative; spasmolytic; treats rheumatism; removes warts and clears the skin.

Jen shen

Ninjin
Panax Ginseng
Ginseng

The crude drug is the root. The red variety is sun dried after having been steamed for about two hours. The white variety is sun dried after the skin has been removed.

PROPERTIES: tonic; stomachic; aids longevity.

Wild ginseng is of higher quality than cultivated ginseng. The plants are at their peak for pharmaceutical use at five or six years of age. The roots are dug in the fall.

Jên tung

Nindo
Lonicera japonica
Honeysuckle

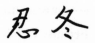

The crude drug is the leaves and stems.

PROPERTIES: antitoxic—discharges poisons; diuretic; hemocathartic; treats syphilitic skin diseases and tumors.

Jên tung chiu (Japanese, Nindoshu), a beverage with the same medicinal properties as the herb, is made by steeping the herb in liquor.

Kan chiang

> Kankyo
> Zingiber officinale
> Steamed ginger

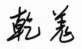

The crude drug is the root which has been steamed and dried.

PROPERTIES: antiemetic; antitussive; warming; analgesic for stomach-aches; stomachic; cardiac stimulant.

Kan ti huang

> Kanjio
> Rehmania glutinosa

The crude drug is the sun dried root.

PROPERTIES: hematopoietic; coagulant; abates thirst; treats heart attacks; relieves burning feet.

Kan ts'ao

> Kanzo
> Glycyrrhiza glabra
> Licorice

The crude drug is the root.

PROPERTIES: expectorant; analgesic; vasodilator; hematopoietic; stomachic; antipyretic; strengthens the spleen and lungs.

Ke Ken, Ke

> Kakon
> Pueraria lobata, P. hirsuta
> Hair grass

The crude drug is the root which has been cut crosswise.

PROPERTIES: diaphoretic; antipyretic; spasmolytic; demulcent for gastrointestinal catarrhs.

Keng mi

> Kobei
> Oryza sativa
> Brown rice

The crude drug is the grain.

PROPERTIES: benefits the lungs and breath; relieves anxiety; abates thirst; checks discharges; warms the viscera; harmonizes the stomach.

K'u shen

　Kujin
　Sophora augustifolia

苦参

The crude drug is the root.

PROPERTIES: antipyretic; diuretic; stomachic; vermicide.

The crude drug is toxic in large doses.

Kua lou jen, Kua lou shih

　Karonin, Karojitsu
　Trichosanthes Kirilowii

瓜呂實

The crude drug is the seeds.

PROPERTIES: antitussive; expectorant.

The seeds are crushed and applied externally to treat skin disease.

Kua lou ken

　Karokon
　Trichosanthes Kirilowii

瓜呂根

The crude drug is the root.

PROPERTIES: antipyretic; nutrient; lactogogue; abates thirst.

The crude drug is applied externally for eczema and skin disease.

Kua lou shih (see Kua lou jen)

Kua tzu, Tung kua tzu

　Togashi
　Benincasa cerifera

瓜子

The crude drug is the seeds.

PROPERTIES: diuretic; discharges pus; antitussive.

Kuei

Kishi

Cinnamonum cassia, C. obtussifolium, C. zeylanicum, C. sieboldi
Cinnamon

The crude drug is the bark.

PROPERTIES: sudorific; analgesic; antipyretic; carminative; stomachic;
regulates stomach and liver temperatures.

Kung mai nieh (see Chiao-i)

Lien ch'iao

Rengyo
Forsythia suspensa
Weeping forsythia

The crude drug is the dried fruit.

PROPERTIES: diuretic; discharges pus; antitoxic; antihelminthic; treats
tumors and scrofula; relieves painful urination; reduces swellings.

Lien tzu

Renshi
Nelumbo nucifera

The crude drug is the seeds.

PROPERTIES: tonic; diuretic; stomachic.

Lung ku

Ryukotsu
Fossilized bone

The crude drug is the powdered fossil.

PROPERTIES: spasmolytic; sedative.

Lung tan

Jigyo
Gentiana macrophylla, G. scabra

The crude drug is the short rhizome and its branched roots.

PROPERTIES: stomachic; analgesic; antipyretic.

Lung tan ts'ao

> Ryutan
> Gentiana scabra
> Rough Gentian

龍胆

The crude drug is rhizome and branching roots.

PROPERTIES: removes excess heat or cold from the bones; treats eye disorders; treats swollen, aching feet and ulcers.

Lung yen jou

> Ryuganniku
> Nephelium Longana

龍眼肉

The crude drug is the dried fruit.

PROPERTIES: tonic; treats insomnia.

Ma huang

> Mao
> Ephedra gerardiana, E. sinica, E. distachya

麻黄

The crude drug is the stalks of the grass.

PROPERTIES: bronchial muscle relaxant; vasoconstrictive; hypertensive; diaphoretic; expectorant; treats coughs and severe bronchitis and inflammation of nasal membranes; relieves fever, blocked ears, retention of urine, sinus headaches, and exudations of eye inflammations.

Ephedrine, the active ingredient in ma huang, is very similar to adrenaline in chemical structure.

Ma jen, Huo ma, Ta ma

> Mashinin
> Cannabis sativa
> Hemp (species)

麻子仁

The crude drug is the seeds.

PROPERTIES: mild laxative; sedative; treats asthma; spasmolytic.

Ma yuen (see I i jên)

Mai men tung

Bakumondo
Ophiopogon ohwii, O. japonicus

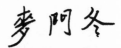

The crude drug is the nodule of the root which has been washed and dried.

PROPERTIES: antitussive; abates thirst; expectorant.

Man ching tzu

Mankeishi
Vitex rotundifolia, V. trifolia

The crude drug is the seeds.

PROPERTIES: antipyretic; cooling; tonic.

Mang ch'ung

Bochu
Tabanus trigonus
Gadfly

The crude drug is the whole fresh or dried body of the insect.

PROPERTIES: anticoagulant; relieves hemostasis; dissolves blood clots; treats paralysis due to blood clots on the brain; employed to prevent paralysis following concussion or stroke.

Mang hsiao

Bosho
$Na_2SO_4H_2O$

The crude drug is the mineral.

PROPERTIES: strong diuretic; strong laxative.

Ming cha

Mokka
Chaenomeles sinensis, Cydonia sinensis
Quince

The crude drug is the dried fruit.

PROPERTIES: diuretic; antitussive.

Mu fang

Boi, Mokuboi
Aristolochia fanchi

木防己

The crude drug is the root.

PROPERTIES: diuretic; analgesic.

Mu hsiang

Mokko
Sanssurea lappa, S. chinensis

木香

The crude drug is the root.

PROPERTIES: stomachic.

Mu li

Borei
Crassostrea giga

牡蠣

The crude drug is the powdered shell.

PROPERTIES: analgesic; abates thirst.

Mu tan pi

Botanpi
Paeonia Moutan, P. suffruticosa
Tree peony

牡丹皮

The crude drug is the bark of the root, after the xylem is removed.

PROPERTIES: vasotonic; analgesic; antiphlogistic.

Mu t'ung

Mokutsu
Akebia quinata

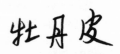

The crude drug is the xylem which has been cut crosswise.

PROPERTIES: diuretic; treats edema, nephritis, and gonorrhea.

Mu t'ung is rich in potassium. It contains as much as 30 percent by weight. The diuretic action of the crude drug may be in part attributed to this factor.

Niu hsi

Goshitsu
Achryanthes fanriei

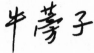

The crude drug is the root.

PROPERTIES: vasotonic; diuretic; emmenagogue.

Niu p'ang tze

Goboshi
Arctium Lappa
Great burdock

The crude drug is the root.

PROPERTIES: antitoxic; antipyretic; laxative; diuretic; reduces swelling and soothes ulcers; relieves skin rashes.

Pai chih

Byakyshi
Horgelica dahurica

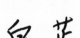

The crude drug is the root.

PROPERTIES: analgesic; expectorant.

P'ai shao (see Shao yao)

Pai shu

Byakujutsu
Attractylodes chinensis, A. japonica, A. lancea

The crude drug is the peeled root.

PROPERTIES: expectorant; tonic; diuretic; antisudorific; stomachic; antiemetic; antidiarrhetic; treats fistulas.

Pan hsia

Hange
Pinellia ternata

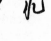

The crude drug is the tuber which has been washed and scoured with sand to remove the exoderm and then sun dried.

PROPERTIES: antiemetic; antitussive; expectorant; treats asthma.

The exoderm contains a substance which is severely irritating to mucous membranes.

Pei mu

    Baimo
    Fritillaria thunbergii
    Imperial Fritillary

The crude drug is the bulb which has been peeled, dusted with lime, and dried.

PROPERTIES: antipyretic; antitussive; expectorant; discharges pus; dumulcent for inflamed throat; treats rheumatism; treats eye infections.

The raw bulb contains a poison that attacks the heart; once cooked, however, its toxicity is destroyed.

Pin lang tzu

    Binroshi
    Areca Catechu

The crude drug is the dried fruit.

PROPERTIES: stomachic; antihelminthic; laxative; relieves swelling.

P'u ho, Po ho

    Hakka
    Mentha arvensis
    Mint (species)

The crude drug is the stalks and leaves.

PROPERTIES: diaphoretic; antipyretic; stomachic; diuretic.

P'u kung ying, Ching p'o po, Chung p'o po

    Hokoei
    Taraxacum officinale
    Dandelion

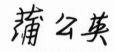

The crude drug is the whole dried plant.

PROPERTIES: lactogogue; stomachic; diuretic; cholagogue; treats skin ulcers.

A paste of the crushed leaves is applied externally to treat boils.

San pai pi

   Sohakuhi
   Mons alba, M. multicaulis

The crude drug is the bark of the root minus the cork layer.

PROPERTIES: diuretic; antitussive; laxative; antiphlogistic.

The crude drug is steeped in liquor to make a beverage that promotes longevity.

Shan chu yü

   Sanshuyu
   Cornus officinalis
   Cornelian cherry

The crude drug is the dried drupes from which the seeds have been removed before drying.

PROPERTIES: tonic; restorative; antitoxic; used to treat senility, lumbago, diabetes, chronic nephritis, and arteriosclerosis.

The dried drupes are steeped in liquor to make a rejuvenative drink.

Shan t'uei (see Ch'an t'uei)

Shan yao, Shu yü

   Sanyaku
   Dioscorea Batatas

The crude drug is the peeled and dried root.

PROPERTIES: tonic; nutrient; antidiarrhetic; abates thirst; treats bed-wetting; relieves night sweating.

Shao yao, P'ai shao

   Shakuyaku
   Paeonia albiflora, P. lactiflora
   Peony root

The crude drug is the root, dug in autumn, which has been washed and dried. The cork layer may or may not be removed.

PROPERTIES: spasmolytic; analgesic for headache, menstrual pain, gastric spasm, and neuralgia; treats afflictions related to pregnancy, childbirth, and gynecopathy.

Shêng chiang

> Shokyo
> Zingiber officinale
> Ginger

The crude drug is the dried rhizome.

PROPERTIES: stomachic; cardiac stimulant.

Sheng ma

> Shoma
> Cimicifuga simplex, C. foetida

The crude drug is the dried rhizome.

PROPERTIES: sudorific; antipyretic; antitoxic; analgesic for headache.

Sheng ti huang

> Shojio
> Rehmania glutinosa

The crude drug is the half-dried root.

PROPERTIES: hematopoietic; coagulant; abates thirst; treats heart attacks; relieves burning feet.

Shih kao

> Sekko
> $CaSO_4 \cdot 2H_2O$
> Gypsum

The crude drug is the mineral.

PROPERTIES: antipyretic; abates thirst.

Shu chiao (see Ch'uan chiao)

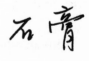

Shu ti huang

Jukujio
Rehmania glutinosa

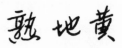

The crude drug is the root which has been steamed and dried. Its color is black.

PROPERTIES: hematopoietic; coagulant; abates thirst; treats heart attacks; relieves burning feet.

Shu yü (see Shan yao)

Shui chih

Suitetsu
Annelida hirudinea
Leech

The crude drug is the whole fresh or dried body of the leech.

PROPERTIES: anticoagulant; relieves hemostasis; dissolves blood clots; treats paralysis due to blood clots on the brain; employed to prevent paralysis following concussion or stroke.

So sha

Shukusha
Amomum xanthiodes

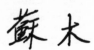

The crude drug is the seeds.

PROPERTIES: stomachic; antiemetic; antidiarrhetic.

Su mu, Su fang mu

Soboku
Caesalpinia Sappan
Sapan wood

The crude drug is wood from this species of tree.

PROPERTIES: coagulant.

Su tzu

Soshi
Perilla frutescens, P. ocymoides

The crude drug is the seeds.

PROPERTIES: antitussive; diuretic; stomachic.

Su yeh

Shisoyo, Shiso
Perilla frutescens

蘇葉

The crude drug is the stems and leaves.

PROPERTIES: stomachic; diaphoretic; antipyretic; antitussive; analgesic.

Suan tsao jen

Sansonin
Zizyphus jujuba (var. spinosa)

酸棗仁

The crude drug is the seeds which have been removed from the drupes.

PROPERTIES: sedative; brings on sleep; benefits the nervous system.

Szu ti

Shitei
Diospyros chinensis, D. Kaki
Calix of persimmon

柿蒂

The crude drug is the dried calix of the common persimmon.

PROPERTIES: spasmolytic; relieves hiccups.

Ta fu p'i

Daifukuhi
Areca Catechu
Palm (species)

大腹皮

The crude drug is the bark.

PROPERTIES: diuretic; stomachic; laxative; vermicide; relieves serious swelling.

Ta huang

Daio
Rheum palmatum, R. corearum
Rhubarb (species)

大黄

The crude drug is the rhizome.

PROPERTIES: laxative; stomachic; treats dropsy, purulent fever, coughs, hoarseness; hypotensive; treats high blood pressure and related heart conditions.

The best quality Ta huang comes from Szechuan and Kansu provinces, but this type of Ta huang is rare and costly. The more common type, Rheum corearum, comes from Yunnan.

Ta ma (see Ma jen)

Tai che shih

Diashaseki
Fe_2O_3
Haematite, Iron ore

The crude drug is the mineral.

PROPERTIES: hematopoietic; coagulant.

Tang kuei

Toki
Angelica acutiloba, A. sinensis, A. polymorpha

The crude drug is the root.

PROPERTIES: tonic; sedative; emmenagogue; hematopoietic; vasotonic; analgesic; hemocathartic; treats hemorrhoids; vasodilator; draws pus from boils.

T'ao jen

Tonin
Prunus Persica
Peach seeds

The crude drug is the seed.

PROPERTIES: analgesic; vasotonic; demulcent for sore throat; antitussive; vasocathartic.

The crude drug is toxic in large doses.

Teng hsin ts'ao

Toshinso
Juncus effusus
Lampwick grass

燈心草

The crude drug is the whole plant.

PROPERTIES: diuretic for kidney disorders.

Ti huang (see also Kan ti huang, Sheng ti huang, Shu ti huang)

Jio
Rehmania glutinosa

地黄

The crude drug is the root.

PROPERTIES: hematopoietic; coagulant; abates thirst; treats heart attacks; relieves burning feet.

The fresh juice is applied externally as a hemostatic.

Ti ku p'i

Jykoppi, Chikoppi
Lycium chinense

地骨皮

The crude drug is the bark of the root.

PROPERTIES: antipyretic; tonic; contains rutin.

Silk bags in which the fruit is crushed are steeped in four times their volume of liquor for two weeks to make a liquor for longevity.

Tiao têng kou

Chodoko, Chotoko
Unsaria rhynchophylla

釣藤鉤

The crude drug is the hooked thorn.

PROPERTIES: spasmolytic; sedative.

T'ien ma

Tenma
Gastrodia elata

天麻

The crude drug is the tuber which has been steamed and dried.

PROPERTIES: tonic; promotes longevity.

T'ien ma is used with Hsiung ch'iung in the preparation of a decoction used to treat headaches accompanied by dizziness.

Ting hsiang

   Choko
   Eugenia caryophyllata
   Cloves

The crude drug is the calyx with the embryo seed attached.

PROPERTIES: stomachic.

Ts'ang chu, Ts'ang shu

   Sojutsu
   Attractylodes chinensis, A. japonica, A. lancea

The crude drug is the unpeeled root.

PROPERTIES: stomachic; diuretic; tonic; expectorant; antiemetic; antidiarrhetic; relieves fistulas.

Tsao

   Daiso
   Zizyphus jujuba (variety inermis)

The crude drug is the drupe which has been sun dried, steamed, and then dried in the shade.

PROPERTIES: tonic; diuretic; corrigent; vasotonic; supports heart and lung functions; dries up excess mucus.

The drupe is used in cooking and is the main ingredient in a popular confection.

Tsê hsieh

   Takusha
   Alisma plantago aquatica, A. plantago orientalis
   Water plantain

The crude drug is the rhizome.

PROPERTIES: diuretic; abates thirst; antidiarrhetic; treats kidney diseases.

Tsung lü yeh

Shuruyo
Trachycarpus excelsus
Coir palm

The crude drug is the leaves.

PROPERTIES: antitoxic; discharges poison; lowers blood pressure.

Tu chung

Tochu
Euonymus tricocarpus, E. ulmoides

The crude drug is the bark.

PROPERTIES: tonic; analgesic; lowers blood pressure.

T'u fu ling

Dobukuryo, Sankirai
Smilax pseudochina

The crude drug is rhizome.

PROPERTIES: antitoxic; discharges poisons and the excess uremic acid
present in humans who consume large quantities of animal flesh;
diuretic; treats syphilitic skin disease and scrofula.

Tu hou

Dokkutsu
Angelica grosseserrata

The crude drug is the root.

PROPERTIES: diaphoretic; analgesic.

Tung kua tzu (see Kua tzu)

Tzu ts'ao

Shikon
Lithospermum officinale, L. erythrorhizon
Groomwell

The crude drug is the root.

PROPERTIES: antipyretic; antitoxic; discharges poison; treats syphilitic skin diseases.

The powdered crude drug is mixed with sesame oil and applied to burns, wounds, eczema, and hemorrhoids.

Wei ling hsien

Ireisen
Clematis terniflora
Virgin's-bower

威靈仙

The crude drug is the root.

PROPERTIES: diuretic; analgesic; promotes circulation.

Wu chu yü

Goshuyu
Evodia rutaecarpa

吳茱萸

The crude drug is the dried fruits.

PROPERTIES: analgesic; diuretic; stomachic.

Wu wei tzu

Gomishi
Schizandra chinensis

五味子

The crude drug is the dried fruits.

PROPERTIES: antitussive; tonic; sedative; nutrient.

Yen hu so

Engosaku
Corydalis ambigua

延胡索

The crude drug is the bulb.

PROPERTIES: analgesic; vasotonic; emmenagogue.

Yin ch'en

Inchinko
Artemisia capillaris
Wormwood

茵陳

The crude drug is the stalks and seeds.

PROPERTIES: diaphoretic; expels heat from lungs; diuretic; cholagogue; treats jaundice; treats headaches and vertigo.

Ying pi

Ohi
Prunus yedoensis
Cherry bark

The crude drug is the bark of the tree.

PROPERTIES: antitoxic; antitussive.

Yu chin

Ukon
Curcuma Longa
Turmeric

The crude drug is the rhizome which has been dried after having been soaked for a while in boiling water.

PROPERTIES: stomachic; emmenagogue; diuretic; hemostatic; used in treating hemoptysis, epistaxis, and hematuria; promotes absorption of oil and vitamin A; increases scotopic vision.

Yüan chih

Ongi
Polygala tenuifolia
Milkwort, Snakeroot, Seneca root

The crude drug is the root.

PROPERTIES: sedative; expectorant; improves vision; improves hearing; treats lapses of memory and poor concentration.

The primary active ingredient in Yüan chih is methylsalicylate.

APPENDIXES

Romanized Japanese-Chinese Index of Teas

Bakumondoto	Mai men tung t'ang
Bofutsushosan	Fang feng t'ung shêng san
Boioghito	Fang yi huang t'ang
Bukukyoin	Fu ling yin
Bushito	Fu tzu t'ang
Byakkoto	Pai hu chia jen shen t'ang
Choijokito	T'iao wei ch'eng ch'i t'ang
Choreito	Chu ling t'ang
Daijokito	Ta ch'eng ch'i t'ang
Daiobotanpito	Ta huang mu tan t'ang
Daisaikokaryukotsuboreito	Ta ch'ai hu chia lung ku mu li t'ang
Daisaikoto	Ta ch'ai hu t'ang
Daiseiryuto	Ta ch'ing lung t'ang
Diaobushito	Ta huang fu tzu t'ang
Eppito	Yüeh pei t'ang
Goreisan	Wu ling t'ang
Goshakusan	Wu chi san
Hachimigan	Pa wei wan
Hangekobokuto	Pan hsia hou p'o t'ang
Hangeshashinto	Pan hsia hsieh hsin t'ang
Hei i san	P'ing wei san
Hochuekkito	Pu chung yi ch'i t'ang
Hokoeito	P'u kung ying t'ang
Inchingoreisan	Yin ch'en wu ling san
Inchinkoto	Yin ch'en kao t'ang
Ishoho	Wei cheng fang
Jijinmeimokuto	Shih shen ming mu t'ang
Jujendaihoto	Shih ch'uan ta pu t'ang

143

Jumihaidokuto	Shih wei t'iao tu t'ang
Junchyoto	Jun ch'ang t'ang
Kakonto	Ke ken t'ang
Kamishoyosan	Chia wei hsiao yao san
Kanbakudaisoto	Kan mai ta tsao t'ang
Kangawagedokuto	Hsing ch'uan chieh tu t'ang
Kanzobushito	Kan ts'ao fu tzu t'ang
Karokijutsuto	Kua lou chih shih t'ang
Karoto	Kua lou t'ang
Keikairengyoto	Ching chieh lien ch'ih t'ang
Keikyososoohshinbuto	Kuei chiang tsao ts'ao hsin fu t'ang
Keimeisan	Chi ming san ch'ia fu ling
Keishibukuryogan	Kuei chih fu ling wan
Keishikaryukotsuboreito	Kuei chih chia lung ku mu li t'ang
Keishikashakuyakuto	Kuei chih chia shao yao t'ang
Keishito	Kuei chih t'ang
Kihito	Kuei p'i t'ang
Kikyoto	Chieh keng t'ang
Kokosan	Hsiang su t'ang
Kuminbinroto	Chiu wei pin lang t'ang
Kyukikyogaito	Hsiung kuei chiao chih t'ang
Makyokansekito	Ma hsing kan shih t'ang
Makoyokukonto	Ma hsing yi kan t'ang
Maobushisaishinto	Ma huang fu tzu hsi hsin t'ang
Maoto	Ma huang t'ang
Mashiningan	Ma tzu jen wan
Mokuboito	Mu fang i t'ang
Ohdoto	Huang tu t'ang
Ohgikenchuto	Huang chü chien chung t'ang
Ohrengedokuto	Huang lien chieh tu t'ang
Otsujito	Yi tzu t'ang
Renjuin	Lien chu t'ang
Richuto	Li chung t'ang
Rikakuto	Li mo t'ang
Rikkosan	Li hsiao san
Ryokankyoninshingeninto	Ling kan chiang wei hsin hsia jen t'ang

Ryokeijutsukanto	Ling kuei shu kan t'ang
Ryutanshakanto	Lung tan hsieh kan t'ang
Saikokaryukotsuboreito	Ch'ai hu chia lung ku mu li t'ang
Saikokeishito	Ch'ai hu kuei chih t'ang
Saikokishikankyoto	Ch'ai hu kuei kan chiang t'ang
Sanmishakosaito	San wei che ku ts'ai t'ang
Sanohshashinto	San huang hsieh hsin t'ang
Sansoninto	Suan tsao jen t'ang
Seinetsugentsuto	Ch'ing je chieh yu t'ang
Senkanmeimokuto	Hsi kan ming mu t'ang
Sesshoin	Che ch'ung yin
Shakanzoto	Chih kan ts'ao t'ang
Shakukanohshinbuto	Shao kan huang hsin fu t'ang
Shakuyakukanzoto	Shao yao kan ts'ao t'ang
Shigyakuto	Szu ni t'ang
Shikumshinto	Szu chün tzu tang
Shimotsuto	Szu wu t'ang
Shinbuto	Chen wu t'ang
Shishihakuhito	Chih tzu pai pi t'ang
Shishikanrento	Chih tzu kan lien t'ang
Shiteito	Szu ti t'ang
Shohangebukuryogan	Hsiao pan hsia fu ling t'ang
Shojokito	Hsiao ch'eng ch'i t'ang
Shokenchuto	Hsiao chien chung t'ang
Shosaikoto	Hsiao ch'ai hu t'ang
Shoseiryuto	Hsiao ching lung t'ang
Soshikokito	Su tzu chiang ch'i t'ang
Teitogan	Ti tang wan
Tokakujokito	Ts'ao ho ch'eng ch'i t'ang
Tokikenchuto	Tang kuei chien chung t'ang
Tokishakuyakusan	Tang kuei t'iao yao san
Tokishigyakukagoshuyukyoto	Tang kuei szu ni chia wu chu yü shêng chiang t'ang
Tsudosanshazenshi	T'ung tao san
Unsei-in	Wen ch'ing yin
Yokuinto	Yi yi jen t'ang
Yokukansan	Yi kan san

Romanized Japanese-Chinese Index of Herbs

Akyo	A chiao
Baimo	Pei mu
Bakumondo	Mai men tung
Binroshi	Pin lang tzu
Bochu	Mang ch'ung
Bofu	Fang feng
Boi, Mokuboi	Mu fang
Borei	Mu li
Bosho	Mang hsiao
Botanpi	Mu tan pi
Bukuryo	Fu ling
Bushi	Fu tzu
Byakujutsu	Pai shu
Byakyshi	Pai chih
Chikoppi (see Jykoppi)	
Chikujo	Chu ku, Chu ju
Chimo	Chih mu
Chinpi	Ch'ên p'i
Chodoko, Chotoko	Tiao têng kou
Choko	Ting hsiang
Chorei	Chu ling
Daifukuhi	Ta fu p'i
Daio	Ta huang
Daiso	Tsao
Diashaseki	Tai che shih
Dobukuryo, Sankirai	T'u fu ling
Dokkutsu	Tu hou
Engosaku	Yen hu so
Gaihaku	Hsieh pai
Gaiyo, Kaiyo	Ai yen
Goboshi	Niu p'ang tze
Gomishi	Wu wei tzu
Goshitsu	Niu hsi
Goshuyu	Wu chu yü

Habu	Chüeh ming tzu
Hakka	P'u ho, Po ho
Hange	Pan hsia
Hokoei	P'u kung ying, Ching p'o po
Inchinko	Yin ch'en
Ireisen	Wei ling hsien
Jigyo	Lung tan
Jio	Ti huang
Jukujio	Shu ti huang
Jykoppi, Chikoppi	Ti ku p'i
Kaika	Huai hua
Kaiso (see Shakosai)	
Kaiyo (see Gaiyo)	
Kakon	Ke Ken, Ke
Kan mi	Hsiao mai
Kanjio	Kan ti huang
Kankyo	Kan chiang
Kanzo	Kan ts'ao
Karokon	Kua lou ken
Karonin, Karojitsu	Kua lou jen, Kua lou shih
Kasseky	Hua shih
Keigai	Ching chieh
Ketsumeishi	Fan hsieh yeh
Kikoko	Chih ka
Kikuka	Chü hua
Kikyo	Chieh keng
Kippi	Chü p'i
Kishi	Kuei
Koboku	Hou p'o, Chung pu
Kobushi	Hsiang fu tzu
Ko-i	Chiao i, Kung mai nieh
Koka	Huang hua, Huang lan hua
Kujin	K'u shen
Kyjitsu	Chih shih
Kyo	Chiang
Kyokatsu	Chiang huo
Kyonin	Hsing jen

Mankeishi	Man ching tzu
Mao	Ma huang
Mashinin	Ma jen, Huo ma, Ta ma
Mokka	Ming cha
Mokko	Mu hsiang
Mokutsu	Mu t'ung
Nindo	Jên tung
Ninjin	Jen shen
Ohbaku	Huang po
Ohdo	Huang tzu
Ohgi	Huang ch'i
Ohgon	Huang ch'in
Ohi	Ying pi
Ohren	Huang lien
Ongi	Yüan chih
Rengyo	Lien ch'iao
Renshi	Lien tzu
Ryuganniku	Lung yen jou
Ryukotsu	Lung ku
Ryutan	Lung tan ts'ao
Saicha	Hsi cha
Saiko	Ch'ai hu
Saishin	Hsi hsin
Sankirai (see Dobukuryo)	
Sanshishi	Chih tzû mien
Sanshuyu	Shan chu yü
Sanshyo	Ch'uan chiao, Shu chiao
Sansonin	Suan tsao jen
Sanyaku	Shan yao, Shu yü
Sekko	Shih kao
Senkyu	Hsiung ch'iung, Chuan hsiung
Senpukuka	Hsuan fu hua
Shakanzo	Chih kan tsao
Shakosai, Kaiso	Che ku ts'ai
Shakuyaku	Shao yao, P'ai shao
Shazenshi	Ch'e chi'en tzu
Shazensho	Che chi'en tsao

Shikon	Tzu ts'ao
Shin-i	Hsin i
Shisoyo, Shiso	Su yeh
Shitei	Szuti
Shitsurishi	Chi li tzu
Shojio	Sheng ti huang
Shokyo	Shêng chiang
Shoma	Sheng ma
Shukusha	So sha
Shuruyo	Tsung lü yeh
Soboku	Su mu, Su fang mu
Sohakuhi	San pai pi
Sojutsu	Ts'ang chu, Ts'ang shu
Soshi	Su tzu
Suitetsu	Shui chih
Takusha	Tsê hsieh
Tenma	T'ien ma
Tochu	Tu chung
Togashi	Kua tzu, Tung kua tzu
Toki	Tang kuei
Tonin	T'ao jen
Toshinso	Teng hsin ts'ao
Uikyo	Huai hsiang
Ukon	Yu chin
Yokuinin	I'i jên, Ma yuen
Zenko	Ch'ien hu
Zentai	Ch'an t'uei, Ch'en t'uei, Shan t'uei

Latin-Chinese Index of Herbs

Achryanthes fanriei	Niu hsi
Aconitum Carmichaeli, A. fanriei, A. Fischeri	Fu tzu
Akebia quinata	Mu t'ung

Alisma plantago aquatica, A. plantago orientale	Tse hsieh
Allium ascallonicum	Hsieh pai
Amomum xanthiodes	So sha
Anemarrhena asphodeloides	Chih mu
Angelica acutiloba, A. sinensis, A. polymorpha	Tang kuei
Angelica grosseserrata	Pu hou
Annelida hirudinea	Shui chih
Arctium Lappa	Niu p'ang tze
Areca Catechu	Pin lang tzu
Areca Catechu	Ta fu p'i
Aristolochia fanchi	Mu fang
Artemisia capillaris	Yin ch'en
Artemisia princeps, A. vulgaris, A. capillaris	Ai yen
Asarum heterotropoides, A. Sieboldi	Hsi hsin
Astragalus mongholicus, A. membranaceus, A. hoantschy	Huang ch'i
Attractylodes chinensis, A. japonica, A. lancea	Ts'ang shu
Attractylodes chinensis, A. japonica, A. lancea	Pai shu
Benincasa cerifera	Kua tzu, Tung kua tzu
Bupleurum falcatum	Ch'ai hu
Caesalpinia Sappan	Su mu, Su fang mu
Cannabis sativa	Ma jen, Hou ma, Ta ma
Carthamus tinctorius	Huang hua, Huang lan hua
$CaSO_4 \cdot 2H_2O$	Shih kao
Cassia Tora, C. obtusifolia, C. angustifolia	Chüeh ming tzu
Cassia Tora, C. obtusifolia, C. angustifolia	Fan hsieh yeh
Chaenomeles sinensis, Cydonia sinensis	Ming cha
Chrysanthemum moriflorium, C. sinense	Chu hua
Cimicifuga simplex, C. foetida	Sheng ma

Cinnamonum cassia, C. obtusifolium, C. Zeylanicum, C. Sieboldi	Kuei
Citrus aurantium, C. nobilis	Chih shih
Citrus leiocarpa, C. nobilis	Chu p'i
Citrus unshui, C. nobilis	Ch'ên p'i
Clematis terniflora	Mu t'ung
Coix lacryma jobi	I i jên, Ma yuen
Collinite, Kasan aluminum	Hua shih
Coptis japonica, C. sinensis	Huang lien
Cornus officinalis	Shan chu yü
Corydalis ambigua	Yen hu so
Crassostrea giga	Mu li
Curcuma longa	Yü chin
Cyperus rotundus	Hsiang fu tzu
Digenea simplex	Che ku ts'ai
Dioscorea Batatas	Shan yao, Shu yü
Diospyros chinensis, D. Kaki	Szu ti
Ephedra gerardiana, E. sinica, E. distachya	Ma huang
Equus Asinus	A chiao
Eugenia caryophyllata	Ting hsiang
Euonymus tricocarpus, E. ulmoides	Tu chung
Evodia rutaecarpa	Wu chu yü
Foeniculum vulgare	Huai hsiang
Forsythia suspensa	Lien ch'iao
Fritillaria Thunbergii	Pei mu
Gardenia jasminoides	Chih tzû mien
Gastrodia elata	T'ien ma
Gentiana macrophylla, G. scabra	Lung tan
Gentiana scabra	Lung tan ts'ao
Glycyrrhiza glabra	Chih kan ts'ao
Glycyrrhiza glabra	Kan ts'ao
Graptopsaltria nigrofuscata	Ch'an t'uei, Ch'en t'uei or Shan t'uei
Grifola umbellata	Chu ling

Hordeum vulgare	Chiao i
Horgelica dahurica	Pai chih
Inula britannica	Hsuan fu hua
Juncus effusus	Teng hsin ts'ao
Ledebouriella seseloides	Fang feng
Ligusticum Wallichii, Cnidium officinale	Hsiung ch'iung, Chuan hsiung
Lithospermum officinale, L. erythrorhizon	Tzu ts'ao
Lonicera japonica	Jên tung
Lycium chinense	Ti ku p'i
Magnolia denudata	Hsin-i
Magnolia officinalis	Hou p'o, Chung pu
Mentha arvensis	P'u ho, Po ho
Mons alba, M. multicaulis	San pai pi
Na_2SO_4 n H_2O	Mang hsiao
Nelumbo nucifera	Lien tzu
Nephelium longana	Lung yen jou
Notoplerygium incisum	Chiang huo
Ophiopogon ohwii, O. japonicus	Mai men tung
Oryza sativa	Keng mi
Pachyma cocos	Fu ling
Paeonia lactiflora, P. albiflora	Shao yao, P'ai shao
Paeonia Moutan, P. suffruticosa	Mu tan pi
Panax Ginseng	Jen shen
Perilla frutescens	Su yeh
Perilla frutescens, P. ocymoides	Su tzu
Peucedanum dicursivum	Ch'ien hu
Phellodendron amurense	Huang po
Pinellia ternata	Pan hsia
Plantago asiatica, P. major	Ch'e chi'en tsao
Plantago asiatica, P. major	Ch'e chi'en tzu
Platycodon grandiflorum	Chieh keng
Polygala tenuifolia	Yuan chih

Prunus Armeniaca	Hsing jen
Prunus Persica	T'ao jen
Prunus yedoensis	Ying pi
Puccina corticoides	Chu ku, Chu ju
Pueraria lobata, P. hirsuta	Ke ken, Ke
Rehmannia glutinosa	Kan ti huang
Rehmannia glutinosa	Sheng ti huang
Rehmannia glutinosa	Shu ti huang
Rehmannia glutinosa	Ti huang
Rheum palmatum, R. corearum	Ta huang
Rheum undalatum (haematite)	Tai che shih
Sanssurea lappa, S. chinensis	Mu hsiang
Schizandra chinensis	Wu wei tzu
Schizonepeta tennuifolia	Ching chieh
Scutellaria baicalensis	Huang ch'in
Smilax pseudochina	T'u fu ling
Sophora angustifolia	K'u shen
Sophora japonica	Huai hua
Tabanus trigonus	Mang ch'ung
Taraxacum officinale	P'u kung ying
Thea sinensis	Hsi cha
Trachycarpus excelsus	Tsung lü yeh
Trichosanthes Kirilowii	Kua lu jen, Kua lu shih, Kua lu ken
Triticum vulgare	Hsiao mai
Ulex (species)	Chi li tzu
Unsaria rhynchophylla	Tiao teng kou
Vitex rotundifolia, V. trifolia	Man ching tzu
Zanthoxylum piperitum	Ch'uan chiao, Shu chiao
Zingiber officinale	Chiang
Zingiber officinale	Chin chiang
Zingiber officinale	Kan chiang
Zingiber officinale	Shêng chiang
Zizyphus jujuba	Suan ts'ao jen
Zizyphus jujuba	Tsao

Bibliography

Academy of Traditional Chinese Medicine
An Outline of Chinese Acupuncture
Peking: Foreign Languages Press, 1975

Austin, Robert, and Ueda, Koichiro
Bamboo
New York: Walker/Weatherhill, 1970

Braun, R.
List of Medicines Exported from Hangkow and other Yangtze Ports
Shanghai: Inspector General of Customs, 1909

Chang, Chung-yuan
Creativity and Taoism
New York: Harper and Row, 1970

China National Native Produce and Animal By-Product Import and Export
Corporation
Chinese Patent Medicines
Tientsin: n.d.

Fairservis, Walter A. Jr.
The Origins of Oriental Culture
New York: New American Library, 1959

Fullard, Howard (ed.)
China in Maps
London: George Phillips and Sons, 1968

Goodrich, L. Carrington
A Short History of the Chinese People
New York: Harper and Row, 1959

Grousset, René
The Rise and Splendor of the Chinese Empire
Berkeley: University of California Press, 1959

Hashimoto, M.
Japanese Acupuncture
New York: Liveright, 1968

Huard, Pierre, and Wong, Ming
Chinese Medicine
New York: McGraw-Hill, 1968

Jen Yu-ti
A Concise Geography of China
Peking: Foreign Languages Press, 1964

Kariyone, Tatsuo
Atlas of Medicinal Plants
Osaka: Takeda Chemical Industries, 1971

Kendal, Carl
"Magic Herbs: the Story of Chinese Medicine"
China Journal, XVI, No. 6 (June 1932)

Lasagua, Louis
"Herbal Pharmacology and Medical Therapy in The People's Republic of China"
Annals of Internal Medicine, LXXXIII (1975), pp. 887–893

Lavier, J.
Points of Chinese Acupuncture
Northamptonshire: Health Science Press, 1965

Li, C. P.
Chinese Herbal Medicine
Washington, D.C.: U.S. Department of Health, Education and Welfare, 1974

Matthews, R. H.
A Chinese-English Dictionary
Shanghai: China Inland Mission and Presbyterian Mission Press, 1931

Morse, William R.
Chinese Medicine
New York: Paul B. Hoeber, 1934

Needham, Joseph
Science and Civilization in China
Cambridge: Cambridge University Press

Palos, Stephan
The Chinese Art of Healing
New York: Herder and Herder, 1971

Porkert, Manfred
The Theoretical Foundations of Chinese Medicine: Systems of Correspondence
Cambridge, Mass.: M.I.T. Press, 1974

Read, Bernard E.
Chinese Materia Medica: Animal Drugs
Peiping: Peking Natural History Bulletin, 1931 (reprint)

Read, Bernard E.
Chinese Materia Medica: Avian Drugs
Peiping: Peking Natural History Bulletin, 1931–1932 (reprint)

Read, Bernard E.
Chinese Materia Medica: Dragons
Peiping: Peking Natural History Bulletin, 1931–1932 (reprint)

Read, Bernard E.
Chinese Materia Medica: Turtles and Shellfish Drugs
Peiping: Peking Natural History Bulletin, 1937 (reprint)

Read, Bernard E.
Chinese Materia Medica: Fish Drugs
Peiping: Peking Natural History Bulletin, 1939 (reprint)

Read, Bernard E.
Chinese Medicinal Plants: From the Pen Ts'ao Kang Mu, 3rd ed.
Peiping: Peking Natural History Bulletin, 1936 (reprint)

Read, Bernard E.
Famine Foods: Listed in the Chiu Huang Pon Ts'ao
Shanghai: Henry Lester Institute of Medicinal Research, 1946

Read, Bernard E.
"Insects Used in Chinese Medicine"
Journal N. C. Royal Asiatic Society, LXII (1940), pp. 22–32

Read, Bernard E., Lee Wei Yung, and Ch'eng Jih Kuang
Shanghai Foods
Shanghai: Chinese Medical Association, 1937

Read, B. E., and Pak, C.
A Compendium of Minerals and Stones Used in Chinese Medicine
Peiping: Peking Natural History Bulletin, 1936 (reprint)

Smith, F. Porter, and Stuart, G. A.
Chinese Medicinal Herbs
San Francisco: Georgetown Press, 1973

Toguchi, Masaru
Oriental Herbal Wisdom
New York: Pyramid, 1973

U.S. Department of Health, Education and Welfare
A Barefoot Doctor's Manual
Washington, D.C.: U.S. Department of Health, Education and Welfare, 1975

Veith, Ilza (trans.)
The Yellow Emperor's Classic of Internal Medicine (Huang Ti Nei Ching)
Berkeley: University of California Press, 1966

Wallnofer, Heinrich, and Von Rottausher, Anna
Chinese Folk Medicine
New York: Bell, 1965

Welch, Holmes
Taoism: The Parting of the Way
Boston: Beacon Press, 1951

Wilhelm, Hellmut
Change: Eight Lectures on the I Ching
New York: Harper & Row, 1960

Wilhelm, Richard
The I Ching
Princeton, N.J.: Princeton University Press, 1950

Wong, K. Chi Min, and Wu Lien-teh
History of Chinese Herbal Medicine
Shanghai: National Quarantine Service, 1936

Wu Wei-ping
Chinese Acupuncture
Northamptonshire: Health Science Press, 1962

Yashiroda, Kan, and Woodward, Carol H. (eds.)
Handbook of Japanese Herbs and Their Uses
Brooklyn, N.Y.: Brooklyn Botanical Garden, 1968

Japanese Sources

Domei, Yakazu
Kanpo Shoho Kaisetsu (Explanation of Traditional Herbal Medicine)
Osaka: Segensha, 1967

Keisetsu, Otsuka
Kanpo Chiryo No Iten (Treatment by Herbal Medicine with Case Histories)
Tokyo: Nanzando, 1969

Keisetsu, Otsuka; Domei, Yakazu; and Totaro, Shimizu
Kanpo Shinryo Iten (Diagnosis and Treatment of Traditional Chinese Medicine)
Tokyo: Nanzando, 1971

Tsuneo, Nauba
Kanpoyaku Ryumon (Introduction to Herbal Medicine)
Tokyo: Hoikusha, 1969